SUPERHERO NUTRITION

Published by Steve Zim

Photography by Steve Zim, Kennedy Meek, and Kimberly Richey

ISBN 978-164316445-8

Printed in the Unites States of America

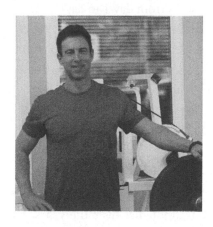

AUTHOR'S NOTE

My name is Steve Zim, and I have been a professional trainer for 29 years. I own a private gym in Culver City, California, called A Tighter U.

I train clients from all walks of life and ages that range from as young as 12 to 93 years old. I am best known for training and creating the nutrition plans for many A-list celebrities and pro and Olympic athletes.

This book started with a Facebook message I received from a producer at BuzzFeed. He had seen a "Celebrity Makeovers" segment I did with Chris Evans for the show *Extra*. I had worked with Chris for 30 days, and had taken him to a superhero level of conditioning. One of the producers at BuzzFeed asked me if I could achieve similar results with two regular people as I had done with Chris.

I said, "game on," and I began to work with a man and a woman (Evan Ghang and Kelsey Impicciche) from BuzzFeed. I had three rules these two online personalities needed to follow to the letter to achieve their goals:

1) **Follow my diet**
2) **Follow my workout**
3) **Follow my cardio program**

BuzzFeed filmed the process from day 1 to day 30. The results were amazing! The YouTube video is called "We Trained Like Superheroes for 30 Days." The video went viral, and it was the fastest video to reach 10 million views produced by BuzzFeed in its history. It was also the #1 trending video on YouTube for 48 hours in January, 2017.

https://youtu.be/okM3OYaBQGg

To date, I've received over 100,000 emails about my videos and the most-asked question I get is: "What was their diet? I want to follow it too!"

I've learned quite a bit about diet over the years. For one thing, almost every diet will work in the beginning. That's why you frequently hear people say, "I'm starting my diet again… " After all, that's when most of these plans work best. People say that every time they want to lose a few pounds. The problem is that bodyweight and body fat are two different things, and they don't keep the weight off. I'll explain why that is later in the book.

My gym has served as a laboratory where I could develop my program to where it is today. Twenty-nine years and thousands of clients later, I want to share my secrets with everyone, because I believe I can change your life and make you feel the best you ever have about yourself.

My nutrition, weight training and cardio programs have been proven to work time and time again. It doesn't matter if you're a regular person looking to get ripped so you can appear in a bathing suit with confidence about how you look, an A-list celebrity who has to play a superhero in three weeks, or a model walking the runway at fashion week in Paris or New York. My program gets quick, long-lasting results. In this book, I'll explain how the nutrition plan works, and why you'll succeed on this plan when all the other nutrition plans have failed you in the past.

Yours in health,

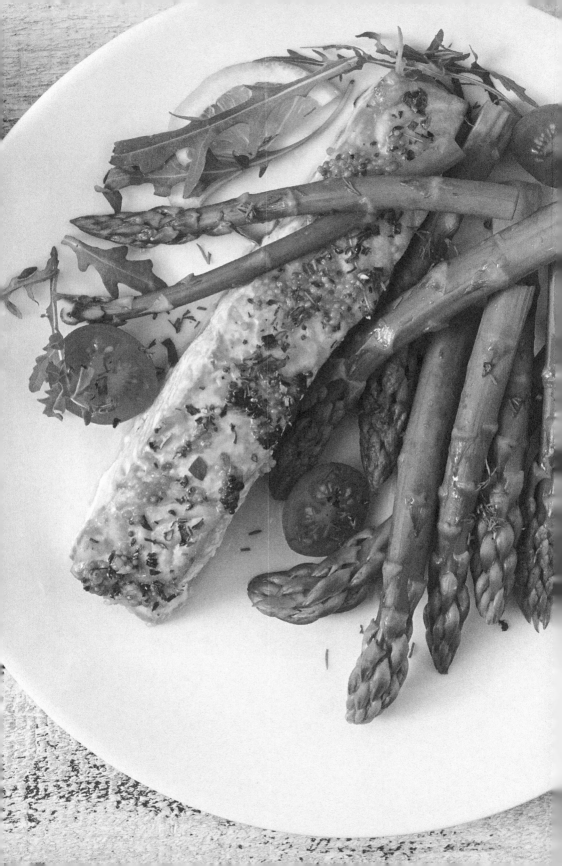

CHAPTER

1

EATING FOR LIFE

A Nutrition Plan that Works. Forever.

have tried many different nutrition programs over the years, both with my clients and for myself. I've achieved a certain amount of success with several of them, especially at first. That's because many of these diets work very well in the short term. But virtually all of them fail over time. Why? Here are a few reasons:

- COMPLIANCE—Many of these programs are challenging to sustain. Sure, if you cut calories super-low, you're going to immediately lose weight. In fact, you may lose quite a bit of weight in a short period. After all, that's what these diets are predicated upon. What happens is you drop water weight and muscle mass very quickly, and you also shed a small amount of fat, although not as much as you probably think. It takes some time to really crank up your body's fat-burning system, and even then it's a slow grind. So, that means much of your quick weight reduction comes from reducing water and muscle mass, things you actually don't want to lose.

- TOO MANY MEALS—Many nutrition programs require you to consume multiple small meals a day, These programs are based on the principle that consuming multiple small meals up your metabolism and help reduce hunger. That's because you have an influx of calories coming into your body many times per day. Some of these diets rely on six or more meals each day and often you never get to consume a proper meal. So, though you're eating all the time, you're never satisfied. All these small meals also put stress on your digestive system, which is hard on the body, an issue I'll explain in more detail later.

- LIMITED FOOD CHOICES—Some of these programs have very limited food choices. Which at first works really well and are easy to do, but within a few days these become monotonous. When you dread your next meal your program is doomed.

There is a better way. And that's where my plan comes in.

HOW "SUPERHERO NUTRITION" WORKS

This book will provide you with my personal program, the one I use with many of my clients. But the beauty of my plan is that if you eat vegan, vegetarian, Paleo, raw food, ketogenic, lactose intolerant, or even if you follow Weight Watchers or any other popular diet, your food choices will work with my system.

Superhero Nutrition is a two-part system:

Part 1: The timing of your meals, workouts and sleep, which is the backbone of the program.

Part 2: What you actually consume every meal.

Part 1 is the most important aspect of my program; if you are eating at the wrong times, no matter how clean your diet is, you won't be able to achieve or maintain your goals. I believe that the way my plan puts your meals together is the most efficient and long-term answer to getting you to lose bodyfat like a superhero.

Do not fear if my foods aren't exactly what you want to eat. My system will guide you to making the perfect choices from the foods you *do* eat. Together we will achieve the goal of getting you in the best shape of your life.

I promise!

HERE'S MY PLAN

I'll go into more detail in Chapter 3, but here are the nuts and bolts of my program.

1) You'll eat 2-3 meals a day. You choose the meals.

2) You'll space your meals 5-6 hours apart with no snacking in between.

3) You *will not* be limited on how much quality food you consume at meals, because you'll have "free" foods, such as salads, to include in your meals.

4) You can follow any other program so long as you adhere to my program's rules. This means you can incorporate diets such as Weight Watchers, South Beach, or lifestyle preferences, such as vegan and vegetarian.

5) I believe you'll have even greater success if you adhere to certain critical guidelines of my program, including:

- my hand-ratio recommendations;
- the glycemic-load principles (which I'll explain later).

In the end, the choice is up to you whether or not you want to follow my food recommendations. The most crucial thing about Superhero Nutrition is my unique timing plan. I'll explain the reasons why this works in the next chapter.

SUPERHERO STORY: The Yo-Yoing Actor

⭐ I started training an actor who was stressed because he had just finished filming a movie and was worried that he wouldn't be ready to play a superhero in his next project in six weeks. So he asked me if he should just eat boiled chicken and salad every day for lunch and dinner and then an apple for breakfast. "I've done it before, and I got in shape," he said.

So I asked him what happened after he stopped eating that way, he laughed and told me he couldn't stop eating carbs and gained 35 pounds quickly afterwards. Then I asked him if he wanted to do it my way and not only get camera-ready but never break down again. He decided to try my program and he's kept the fat off ever since.

WHY OTHER PLANS FAIL OVER TIME

So, you've cut the total number of calories you consume each day. And you've lost 10-20 pounds over the past few weeks. That's good, right?

Yes. That's terrific! But now you have to ask yourself a really difficult question: Can I maintain this program for the rest of my life?

If the answer is no, then you're simply going to gain back the weight you lost. And here comes worse news: You're likely to add even more weight than before you began the diet if you return to your previous eating patterns.

Why? Your metabolism is out of whack because you took in so few calories during those small meals for the past few weeks. While you've successfully lost weight, you've also likely reduced muscle tissue, because your body preferentially burns muscle over stored fat when you're in starvation mode.

Now, when you return to your "normal" eating patterns, your body needs fewer calories per day for activity, and then it will store the excess as bodyfat. It's a vicious cycle that yo-yo dieters often encounter.

Let's say you've fallen into this trap, the way Hollywood stars used to do many years ago—and that continues today, as well. What should you do next? You need to teach your body how to properly manage an appropriate amount of food each day, allowing it to use this fuel to support health and activity without storing it as bodyfat.

That's true whether you've failed on ridiculous diet plans before, or if you've decided to take control of your nutrition program, levels of bodyfat and overall weight for the first time.

SUPERHERO STORY:
The "Hangry" Woman

⭐ I used to train a woman at my gym who was always angry (hangry?), and everything made her upset. Mad about her job, friends and people that got in her way on the street; you name it. So one day she told me how she had not had a good date in over a year. She then explained how she had been on an Intermittent Fasting program for the past year.

"Ah, ha!" I thought to myself, you don't eat for 18 to 20 hours a day then you only have a 4-6-hour window where you can eat whatever you want. She was so unhappy with her nutrition program that it bled into all aspects of her life. Other people in the gym would tell me that they did not want to be around her because she was always in a bad mood. This is no way to go through life just to be in great shape. Your nutrition program should make you feel energetic, happy and not tired and miserable. Mine will help you feel much better. I promise.

WHY SUPERHERO NUTRITION WORKS

Several years ago, I began to investigate other eating strategies that freed me from having to prepare and consume all of those tiny meals with so little satiety. Back in 2007, I wrote a book, The 30-Minute Celebrity Makeover Miracle, in which I recommended that you shouldn't eat for an hour and a half before exercising.

Not eating food for an hour and a half before exercising allows your insulin levels to stabilize. When insulin levels are high, our bodies do not burn fat for energy. That's a simple fact. And the advantage is that the intense calorie demand during training will encourage your body to release fat from storage.

At that time, a light bulb went on over my head. That was the answer! It's all about our bodies' insulin release. Everything else is secondary. I had figured out the solution to permanent fat loss back in 2007, but I hadn't fully understood its importance. That's because I hadn't yet figured out how to fully apply the concept to a sustainable nutrition program.

Now I have.

In the next chapter I'm going to explain all the ins and outs of how insulin works, and how this potent hormone affects you when you follow any nutrition plan. This explains the reasons why virtually all other plans fail in one way or another over time, and why you'll succeed on my program. It's all about timing, and you can integrate any other plan into mine so long as you emphasize timing over calories and foods.

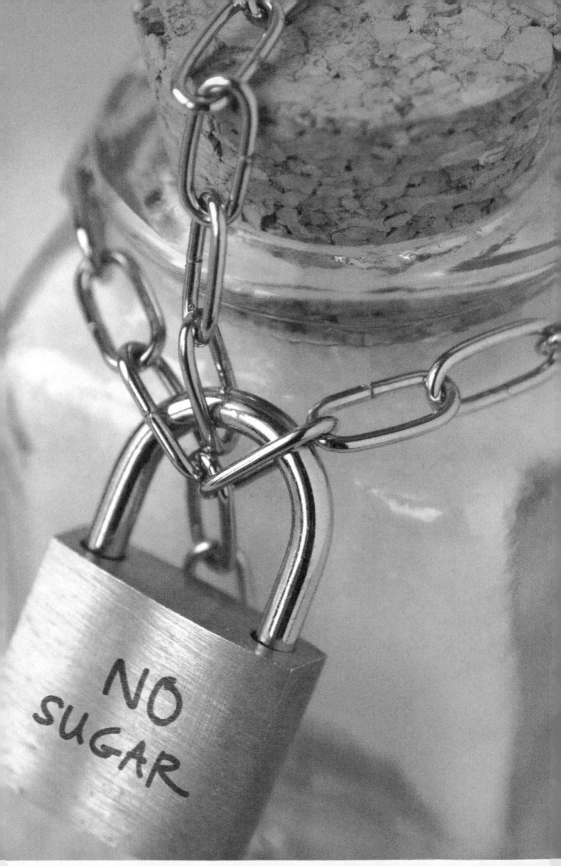

2

THE SWEET SCIENCE

Insulin and Its Impact

So here's the good news: In this chapter, I'm going to go into some detail about how and why my program will help you. The bad news is that this chapter is more complicated than those that follow. It gets into the physiological purposes and actions of insulin.

While this chapter is crucial to understanding how my program works, it's not necessary that you grasp all of the biochemistry and physiology to follow my program. But I feel it's necessary to provide this information because it's based on solid science.

So feel free to skip this chapter and come back to it when you're more interested in WHY it will work rather than WHAT you should do. For the rest of you, put your science hat on and let's learn why my program works right now.

A MOMENT OF SCIENCE: HOW INSULIN WORKS

Insulin is necessary for living. This crucial hormone regulates blood sugar. Here's a step-by-step on how insulin works.

- Insulin is a hormone that is generated in the pancreas. It functions as a transport system.
- When you eat food, it is broken down through a series of steps, from chewing to digestive enzymes. By the time the food you've consumed enters your small intestine, the food is broken down into small enough molecular bits that they can be absorbed through your intestinal wall and into your blood stream.
- Once the nutrients have entered your blood stream, your pancreas delivers insulin to aid in delivery of these nutrients to where it perceives they are needed.

- Most people think insulin is ONLY triggered by consuming carbohydrates, but the truth is that insulin is released when we eat almost anything. Fiber and water are the only things we consume that do not trigger release of insulin. In fact consuming fiber mitigates the release of insulin because it slows entry of other foods into your system.
- Carbohydrates and sugary foods cause your blood-sugar levels to rise. When your blood-sugar levels are high, the pancreas kicks in, releasing insulin to bring your blood sugar down.
- Insulin moves the sugar in your blood to your liver and muscles to use blood glucose as a source of energy. But both your liver and muscles have a limited amount of storage, so any leftover blood sugar is then transported by insulin to be stored as bodyfat.
- Protein does not typically cause a spike in blood sugar, but it does (unexpectedly) cause a rise in insulin secretion. The insulin spike from eating protein lasts about the same amount of time as the spike from eating carbs. Even fats, like trans and saturated fats cause insulin release. So what does this mean?
- To boil it down, your body will not readily burn bodyfat until your body stops releasing insulin. You CANNOT burn stored fat for energy when your body is releasing insulin.

Every time we eat, our body goes through this process. Depending on the quantity and content of what you eat, insulin levels can remain elevated for as long as four hours after your meal. When insulin levels are elevated, your body burns glucose rather than stored fat, and your body can convert everything that enters your body to glucose, including protein and dietary fats.

INSULIN AND DIABETES: TYPE 1 AND TYPE 2

Insulin is necessary for living. This crucial hormone regulates blood sugar. Type 1 diabetics cannot produce insulin, and they must inject it frequently to survive, constantly monitoring their blood-sugar levels.

It's important that every single one of us understands the impact of insulin on our lives so that we make healthy nutrition choices. After all, we now have a type 2 diabetes epidemic in our country. The difference between type 1 diabetes and type 2 is this: Type 1 diabetics don't produce insulin, while type 2 diabetics don't

respond to insulin. Type 2 diabetes is a "lifestyle" disease, caused by poor ⌐
tion habits and lack of exercise.

You may not believe this fact—it's really shocking—but more than 100 milli⌐
Americans suffer from type 2 diabetes or its precursors. That's one out of three ⌐
everyone who lives in this country!

This epidemic is caused by what we choose to eat, when we consume it, and how
much we take in. While type 1 diabetes must be controlled medically, type 2 diabetes is avoidable and/or reversible so long as you are not terribly ill from this lifestyle
disease and you're willing to follow a sound nutrition and workout regimen.

Following my guidelines will not only help you reduce bodyfat, but they
will also help prevent this life-
style disease.

INSULIN SENSITIVITY VS. RESISTANCE

Insulin sensitivity is the rela-
tionship between how much
insulin is needed to lower
blood sugars in your body
with how much you need to
drive healthy physiological
digestive processes.

When you consume the
proper foods, your body
releases a modest amount
of insulin. And when you
take in these foods at the
right times of day (with
the proper amount of time
between meals), insulin helps
promote muscle building

SUPERHERO STORY: Carbs? Sure!

⭐ When the makeover people from BuzzFeed first sat down with me so I could explain my program to them they were a little surprised. They expected me to tell them horror stories of how I got Chris Evans in shape in 4 weeks after they saw the makeover piece I did with him on *EXTRA*. They expected they'd never be able to eat another carb and that they'd be per-forming five hours of cardio and training hard for another five hours every day.

After I went over everything with them they were completely relieved and excited at the same time. They believed they could achieve their goals and sustain them after we were done. To me, it's all about being able to keep what you worked for and making your nutrition plan as easy as possible.

when you train with weights without driving calories you've consumed to fat storage. If you're following the rules I lay out in the next chapter, then your body will
be insulin sensitive, helping you achieve your fat-loss and muscle-building goals.

wever, if you just consume whatever you want whenever you want, then
re setting your body up to become insulin resistant. This is the condition
at creates type 2 diabetes and its precursors, which 100-plus million Americans
lready suffer from.

Insulin resistance is caused by consuming the wrong foods at the wrong time
and in large quantities over a long period. Eventually, your cells stop responding
to the normal flood of insulin you're unleashing by consuming unhealthy foods.
Then, your pancreas responds by releasing even more insulin. This additional
insulin doesn't drive calories to healthy processes, of course. Instead, it takes the
food you're consuming to storage as bodyfat.

But, equally significantly, the large wash of insulin is training your muscle cells
not to accept the benefits of insulin. This is particularly true if you're not stimu-
lating these cells through exercise. This tandem of consuming the wrong foods at
the wrong time in large quantities coupled with too little exercise is what causes
people to develop type 2 diabetes.

Let me provide an example to better explain insulin resistance: Think of your
body as a guy who never drinks, but then gets fairly drunk when he takes one stiff
drink. And he likes it, so he starts drinking more and more. Eventually, he doesn't
even feel the first drink, so he takes in more and more to get that buzz.

When you're taking in insulin-spiking foods every 2-3 hours, you're
undermining the benefits of insulin while increasing the negative effects.
You're shortening your "Burn Zone" (a term I'll explain in the next chapter),
and you're simultaneously becoming more resistant to insulin's benefits.

WHAT'S THE PLAN? LEARN TO USE INSULIN

I've created my nutrition plan to help you take control of your insulin levels.
Remember, insulin is a hormone that directly affects fat storage. If you learn
how to monitor, regulate and control insulin, it can actually break down fat
and build muscle for you.

It's not just about carbs. We have spent years believing carbs are the
primary problem, but they are a catalyst, rather than the only culprit. My
plan shows you how to mitigate hunger, break cravings, and build muscle all
while burning stored body fat.

The key is to know how foods affect insulin and learn to reduce insulin spikes. For instance, **if you eat three moderate meals of lean protein, unprocessed carbs, and fats, you will reduce the duration of your insulin spikes.**

Remember that.

FIND YOUR SET POINT

Everybody has a "set point," a place their body naturally slides to in terms of the amount of calories they burn before additional intake goes to fat storage. It's a challenge to move that set point and even tougher to keep it elevated.

Maybe you worked hard to lose five pounds, but then it seems like one night out is all it takes to pack back on those pounds. My program helps you change your set point, allowing you to maintain this new level where you burn fat more readily while holding and building muscle.

The first step is being absolutely vigilant about what you put in your body and when. Remember not all calories are created equal. If you eat 1,500 calories of ice cream a day, your body will look much different than if you eat 1,500 calories of eggs, fish, chicken, vegetables, and greens. Certain calories cause our bodies to store more bodyfat, while other calories cause certain hormones to secrete at higher levels than others.

I will prepare your body to get the most out of your workouts by placing you in the Burn Zone.

I'll explain how you can utilize your bodyfat to power your day rather than relying on glucose, which not only keeps your fat in storage, but packs more in, regardless of how much or little you're consuming.

When you're taking in insulin-spiking foods every 2-3 hours, you're undermining the benefits of insulin while increasing the negative effects. You're shortening your Burn Zone, and you're simultaneously becoming more resistant to insulin's beneficial effects.

SUGAR IS YOUR ENEMY

Consuming even small amounts of processed sugar make it difficult to lose bodyfat. Red meat and sugar together can elevate your insulin levels for up to four hours after consumption. While red meat provides health advantages, you should avoid all foods with processed sugar. Here's why sugar is the enemy.

Processed sugar, generally sucrose (table sugar) contains a large amount of glucose; it's half glucose and half fructose (fruit sugar). Neither of these types of sugar is healthy. Glucose causes blood hyperglycemia (high blood sugar in our body). Fructose can cause fatty liver and lead to insulin resistance, which is why high-fructose corn syrup is such a terrible additive to foods.

When you have large amounts of glucose in your blood, your pancreas sounds the alarm and releases a large amount of insulin to combat it. Insulin moves glucose into fat and muscle tissue. But insulin often overreacts to an influx of sugar, which causes your blood sugar to drop below normal levels, creating the condition called hypoglycemia.

This low level of blood sugar then makes you hungry, causing you to reach for unhealthy snacks and, even, healthy foods that you shouldn't consume at this time. But hypoglycemia particularly drives your craving for sugar or other fast-digesting carbs.

You feel good when you're eating sugar or other fast-digesting carbs, but soon afterwards you feel tired or hungry, and so you eat them again to feel more energized. And then this cycle repeats, over and over. That's what drives your body to pack on pounds of fat and feel more lethargic, never mind the long-term consequences such as diabetes, heart disease and cancer, all of which excess consumption of sugar is directly linked to. If you want to lose bodyfat and get healthier, then you need to cut out processed sugar, especially high-fructose corn syrup. End of story.

AVOID CRASH-AND-BURN DIETS

Here's another problem: Crash diets cause you to lose muscle mass, which depletes your ability to lose bodyfat. That's because you're reducing the effectiveness of muscle tissue to burn calories. Muscle cells are essentially tiny engines that burn calories, and so you want to increase them, not reduce them. That's true regardless of how much weight you're losing or how quickly. When you have less muscle, your body learns to conserve energy by slowing down your metabolism.

My mantra is the more lean muscle you have the higher your metabolism becomes because your body burns calories to maintain that muscle. Lose the muscle and your metabolism drops, making it more likely your body will hold onto (or add) bodyfat.

Maintaining or adding muscle is how you lose bodyfat. Encouraging insulin release at the proper times is crucial to this. After all, insulin is also an anabolic (muscle-building) hormone, and it stimulates protein synthesis.

I know I started this chapter by saying that elevated insulin levels are detrimental to burning fat. But it's equally important that you understand that insulin, when properly managed, is better than steroids at building muscle. In fact, many bodybuilders inject insulin at specific times of day to over-emphasize this effect. By the way, that's a TERRIBLE, potentially deadly, idea. Never do that.

But here is how you can get the most from beneficial insulin release. Think of this hormone as a transport system that drops off its passengers at three different locations, based on signaling. Your goal is to prioritize these through what and when you eat.

1) Insulin drives nutrients to muscle tissue. That's your goal when you're working out. Insulin supports recovery and muscle growth.

2) Insulin drives nutrients to your liver. This can be beneficial because it helps convert what you've consumed into what your body needs most at this time.

3) Insulin drives nutrients to fat storage. This is, exactly, what you want to avoid. They key is to avoid consuming foods that encourage insulin release when they don't support building muscle and fat loss.

INSULIN: USE IT, DON'T ABUSE IT

Since our bodies have this built in transport system, I want you to learn to use it to your advantage. You'll see this process at work in my BuzzFeed videos, such as "We Trained Like Superheroes For 30 Days," or "We lost 22% Body Fat In 6 Weeks," plus many others.

I supplement my program with branched-chain amino acids (BCAAs) from Hollywood Supps. BCAAs help promote muscle gain and fat loss. The reason I choose Hollywood Supps BCAAs is they are pure without other ingredients that will spike your insulin excessively.

Let me explain how this works. I have my clients take the recommended amount of BCAAs right before and after their workouts (I recommend leucine 1,600 mg, isoleucine 800 mg, valine 800 mg, all free form).

Timing is essential, as with everything else in my program. These amino acids act as carriers that assist your muscles in synthesizing other amino acids needed for building muscle. BCAAs cause a deliberate slight spike in the release of insulin, which then pushes the amino acids straight into your muscles.

BCAAs are both anabolic and anticatabolic (they promote muscle gain and prevent protein breakdown/muscle loss). BCAAs cause a significant increase in protein synthesis and help in the release of growth hormone and insulin. They also help maintain good testosterone-to-cortisol ratios.

In a recent study published in the *Nutritional Journal of Medicine*, researchers concluded that catabolism of muscle tissue can be reduced by supplementing with BCAAs. The researchers concluded that if the anabolic phase is greater than the catabolic phase, then improvement in muscle strength and size will take place.

Other studies have shown that BCAAs cause exactly that and point directly to the reason why they are so effective in helping our bodies get lean. Muscle burns approximately 3 to 4 times the amount of calories that fat does just to

THE DAILY BURN ZONE:

Here's how you can understand the Burn Zone, and visualize when you're in it... and when you're not. Keep in mind that insulin typically spikes for about two hours after you eat a meal, so the Burn Zone doesn't begin until two hours after you complete your meal. You can eat as quickly or slowly as you like, so long as you understand this.

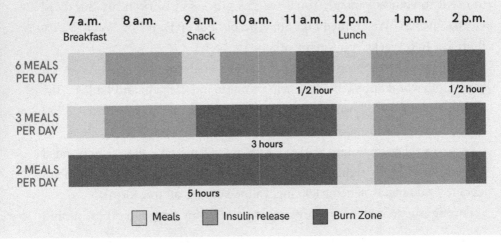

sustain itself. So the more lean muscle mass you have the more calories your body will burn just to sustain that muscle tissue.

This becomes a self-fulfilling prophecy: You tear down muscle tissue when you work out with weights. You do not build muscle when you are lifting; you are actually microscopically tearing muscle. Then, the moment you stop working out your body starts to repair itself and build the muscle. So the nutrition you consume after workouts provides the building blocks you need to add new muscle tissue.

WHAT YOU SHOULD DO

What if I told you that I've discovered a new method of burning fat while eating fewer meals a day? A way to build muscle more readily than ever before while also reducing bodyfat? In addition, you won't have to spend hours on cardio machines. When you follow my Superhero Nutrition program everything falls into place.

All you have to do is follow the 10 rules I explain in the next chapter.

Remember to add in 2 Tbsp. of raw unfiltered apple cider vinegar before each meal to shorten your insulin release window by about 30%. That will significantly increase your Burn Zone, particularly when you're consuming two or three meals per day. When you're consuming 6 meals a day, shortening insulin release is less significant because you're often already eating another meal before you reach the Burn Zone.

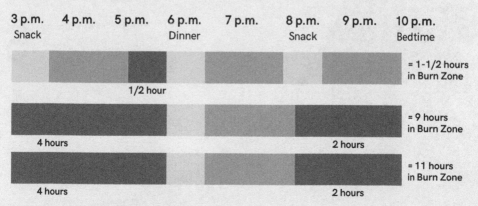

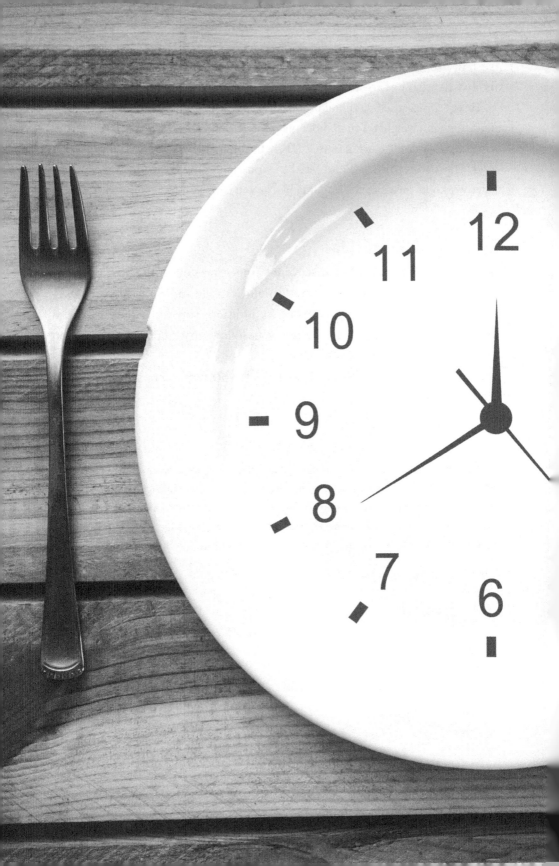

3

10 RULES TO TAKE CONTROL OF YOUR WEIGHT LOSS

An Easy-to-Follow Action Plan

In Chapter 2 you learned about insulin, and the complicated physiological processes it has on fat loss. Those details are important if you want to understand why my program works. Most readers will be more interested in what they need to do to successfully reduce their bodyfat loss, rather than why it works. Whether you understand the science or not, this chapter will give you a plan to put these physical principles into action.

Here I'll explain the 10 rules I want you to follow to put together your program. But I want to make this easy for you to implement. I don't want you to worry about constructing the nuts and bolts of this program yourself. In the chapters following this long one, I'm going to provide detailed guidance on what you need to do every day. I'll provide you with over 50 recipes in Chapters 8-10. They will help you adhere to the 10 rules I'm explaining in detail in this chapter. And I'll also provide a 30-day sample nutrition plan in Chapter 6.

You'll have all the tools you need to make this plan work for you.

So here are my 10 rules for fat loss:

RULE #1: Eat two or three meals per day (with no snacking)

RULE #2: Schedule your meals and your workouts ahead of time every day

RULE #3: Choose the right foods for fat loss

RULE #4: Follow the glycemic load principle

RULE #5: Get your portions right

RULE #6: Take BCAAs before and after your workouts

RULE #7: Drink the right fluids

RULE #8: Follow the rules, but allow yourself a cheat meal

RULE #9: Sleep long and deep

RULE #10: Keep track of your fat-loss results

RULE #1:
EAT TWO OR THREE MEALS PER DAY (WITH NO SNACKING)

This is the most crucial piece of information to understand how you successfully manage your bodyfat levels: **Our bodies can only burn stored fat when our insulin levels are low. Period, end of story.**

Virtually every food you consume encourages insulin release. So, if your goal is to reduce bodyfat, then you need to reduce insulin release. And the best way to do that is to only eat 2-3 times a day, preferably three. Here's what you need to do.

- Eliminate snacking between meals.
- Create longer windows between meals. I recommend spacing your breakfast and lunch apart by at least 5-6 hours. And then you should do the same between lunch and dinner.

This is the most efficient way to keep your insulin levels low for long periods, while also allowing you to take in an appropriate amount of food, nutrients and calories that support daily activity while shedding bodyfat. In addition, you won't go hungry on this plan.

ENTER THE "BURN ZONE"

Once your insulin levels have lowered, your body will be in a state I've dubbed the "Burn Zone." When you lengthen the time you're in a state where your body is not releasing insulin, your body will be encouraged to pull fat from storage to use as fuel for daily activity. If you eat every couple of hours, you'll constantly spike your insulin release. If you do that, you'll either never enter the Burn Zone, or you'll be there only for a short time.

Going for longer periods without consuming meals is more important than the foods you eat. No matter how clean your food choices, you'll have more difficulty burning bodyfat if you're constantly consuming foods or snacks, regardless of their quality. This is why planning the times for your meals is crucial to your success.

When you're in the Burn Zone, your body releases fat from storage, which you can then use to fuel workouts and daily activities. This activity further encourages additional release of stored fat, helping make your Burn Zone more efficient.

In addition to spacing your meals 5-6 hours apart, you should also make sure to consume the last meal before your workout at least 2-3 hours prior to exercise. That's because the additional calorie demands of exercise will further require the release of fat from storage.

When your body is burning fat for energy, you'll begin to see results much more quickly. The positive reinforcement will provide additional motivation to keep following my Superhero Nutrition program. After all, motivation in body transformation only occurs when you begin to see positive changes.

The key is to limit yourself to eating no more than three times a day with no snacking in between. Even healthy foods such as a handful of nuts will undermine the benefits you'll get from the Burn Zone.

KEEP YOUR BEVERAGES SUGAR-FREE

You can drink water, carbonated water (with no sodium or sugar), tea, and coffee between meals. But make sure you don't add anything to these drinks such as cream, sugar or sugar substitutes. Recent research indicates that even no-calorie sugar substitutes likely trigger insulin release. This is due to the fact that these chemicals mimic the activity of sugar in our bodies, which then releases insulin. And that's precisely what you're trying to avoid.

When you make this change, it will take a couple days to get used to it. For people like me who were eating 6-7 times a day, it will take somewhere between 3-7 days to get used to this new eating rhythm. You'll feel pretty hungry—and even sluggish—between meals, but then your body will adapt. Keep in mind that you're teaching your body to use fat, not sugar, to power you through your day.

As you get used to eating three times a day, you'll start having more energy. You'll start to experience greater focus with all of your daily tasks, including your workouts. My nutrition program will help you become a fat-burning, clear-thinking machine!

YOUR ACTION PLAN

▶ Eat only 2-3 meals a day
▶ Space each meal at least 5 hours after the previous
▶ Plan your workouts after you've gone at least 2 hours without eating

RULE #2:
SCHEDULE YOUR MEALS AND WORKOUTS AHEAD OF TIME EVERY DAY

It's important that you get your day started correctly from the get-go. That means you need to plan your first meal, and get up early enough that you can consume your other meals within a 5-6 hour window without waiting until late at night for your dinner (Unless you like to eat late at night, which still works, but that's up to you.)

After all, the first meal you eat sets up the timing of every other meal that follows. If you prefer to work out in the morning, then you need to eat your first meal **after** you exercise. Upon waking, your insulin levels are low, and your body is ready to burn fat. That's because you've gone about 12 hours since your dinner the night before. This guarantees a low level of insulin in a healthy person. Before or during your workout, you can drink black coffee, and you can even add up to a tablespoon of low-fat milk, but, again, don't add sugar or sugar substitutes.

You can add milk from any source (e.g., cow, almond, soy, etc.), so long as the amount you include does not exceed 10 calories. Read labels carefully to understand what you're adding to make certain you're not encouraging insulin release, which will prevent you from burning bodyfat.

Also, drink at least one eight-ounce glass of water before you start your workout to make sure you're properly hydrated before training. Then consume a total of two liters of water per day. This can vary from person to person, as some people are uncomfortable with water sloshing around in their gut while they train.

On the other hand, if you don't work out in the morning, then you should eat your first meal fairly shortly after waking. This will help you create those long windows between meals. At this point, you also need to figure out when you're going to have your lunch (at least 5 hours later), and when you're going to have your dinner (at least 5 hours after that). And then your workouts need to come at least 2 hours (if not 3) after one of these later meals. Plan accordingly.

THREE-MEAL-A-DAY SCHEDULES

Here are four examples of how to put your three-meal-a-day schedule together with a workout. Of course, you have a lot of flexibility with timing based on your personal needs, schedules and the time of day you prefer (or are able) to work out. Feel free to make adjustments to these examples based on your schedule.

Workout upon rising:
WORKOUT: 7 a.m.
BREAKFAST: 8:30 a.m.
LUNCH: 1:30 p.m.
DINNER: 7:30 P.M.

Workout after breakfast
BREAKFAST: 7 a.m.
WORKOUT: 10 a.m.
LUNCH: 1 p.m.
DINNER: 7 p.m.

Workout after lunch:
BREAKFAST: 7 a.m.
LUNCH: 1 p.m.
WORKOUT: 3:30 p.m.
DINNER: 7 p.m.

Workout after dinner:
BREAKFAST: 7 a.m.
LUNCH: 1 p.m.
DINNER: 6-7 p.m.
WORKOUT: 8-9 p.m.

TWO-MEAL-A-DAY SCHEDULES

If you prefer to skip breakfast or lunch, only taking in two meals a day, then here are three examples of how to put this schedule together. Of course, it's much easier to meet the timing criteria when you consume fewer meals in your daily schedule. I call the first time you eat "first meal," whether that's breakfast or lunch.

Workout upon rising:
WORKOUT: 7 a.m.
FIRST MEAL: 8 a.m.-12 p.m.
DINNER: 7 p.m.

Workout after first meal:
FIRST MEAL: 7 a.m.-12 p.m.
WORKOUT: 3-5 p.m.
DINNER: 6 p.m.

Workout after second meal:
FIRST MEAL: 7 a.m.-12 p.m.
DINNER: 5-7 p.m.
WORKOUT: 7-9 p.m.

Make sure you have a 2-3-hour break (preferably 3) from your last meal to the start of any workout program if you are trying to burn fat. Don't make yourself crazy if you only have a two-hour window from your last meal to the start of your workout session. The reason I prefer the three-hour window is because it guarantees that your release of insulin will be down, and you'll be in the Burn Zone.

And here's one more addition to the rules I lay out in this chapter: **Don't eat beef and carbs at the meal before your workouts.** The reason for this is that the insulin response to eating beef and carbs at the same time can last up to four hours because it digests slowly. While beef prevents you from entering the Burn Zone for several hours, that doesn't mean it's a bad food at other times of day. Later in this chapter, I'm going to address which foods you should consume and those you should avoid based on their glycemic impact.

SCHEDULE FOR NON-WORKOUT DAYS

The schedule on non-workout days is much simpler because you don't have to plan as much to create that 2-3 hour window before your workout where you don't consume a meal. Overall, my preference is that you eat three meals a day rather than two, but I understand that needs for fuel and lifestyle vary from one person to another.

When I eat beef, I like to make it my last meal of the day. By the morning I will start my day in the Burn Zone. You want to be in the Burn Zone for as much of your waking day as possible.

Remember, it's all about timing and what you actually eat is secondary. It's very important but still secondary.

YOUR ACTION PLAN

▸ Schedule your day ahead of time, whether you're training or not that day
▸ Follow my examples in setting up a 5-6 hour window between meals
▸ Create at least a 2-hour window between your last meal and your workout when your primary goal is burning fat
▸ Timing is even more important than food choices

RULE #3:
CHOOSE THE RIGHT FOODS FOR FAT LOSS

What and how much should you eat?

It should come as no shock that these are two different questions. And I'm going to answer them both in detail. First, I'll address food choices before I explain the portions that are right for you. Again, I'm going to make these easy for you. You aren't going to have to count calories or keep track of macronutrient grams so long as you follow my simple rules for food selection and portion control.

Knowing what you should consume on my plan is as much about realizing what you can take in as compared to what you shouldn't. Many foods will sabotage your fat-loss goals regardless of how many calories they contain.

So, here's what you need to know about food selection, which is broken down into macronutrient groups. Macronutrients consist of protein, fats, and carbohydrates.

PROTEIN SOURCES

My nutrition plan includes a list of optimal sources of protein. Some exceptional proteins, which I've included in the "primary proteins" list, are: whey, egg whites, fish, and chicken and turkey breast. These are low-fat, lean proteins that are absorbed most efficiently and used most effectively by your body to support muscle tissue. Some less exemplary proteins, or "secondary proteins," include: highly marbled cuts of beef, sausages, processed meats, cold cuts, duck, goose and lamb. Secondary proteins have higher fat contents, and are absorbed less readily, and I recommend you consume them sparingly.

PRIMARY PROTEIN SELECTION: Almost all lean meats work within the boundaries of my nutrition plan. The key is to avoid all processed meats, as well as meats that are extremely high in fat. When possible, choose grass-fed animal protein and opt for wild fish over farm-raised fish. Farm-raised fish are fed grains and that changes the nutrition value of the fish, reducing the amount of omega-3s and other healthy fats they contain.

PRIMARY PROTEINS

Poultry—skin off
Chicken thigh—skin off
Chicken leg—skin off
Chicken breast—skin off
Chicken wings—skin off
Turkey breast— skin off
Pork tenderloin
Pork chop
Lamb
Beef (lean)
Lean ground beef (85% fat or higher)
Buffalo
Duck
Fish (any)
Shellfish (any)
Eggs
Egg whites
Beef jerky
Milk low fat
Milk non-fat
Cottage cheese (low- or non-fat)
Cheese
Protein powder (whey, egg albumin)
Greek yogurt (plain)

SECONDARY PROTEINS

Highly marbled cuts of beef
Sausages
Any processed meats
Cold cuts (prepacked and processed)
Goose
Any form of fried protein

VEGAN/VEGETARIAN PROTEINS

Legumes

* Greens don't contain all the amino acids you need, but pairing them with beans and legumes can help make them complete with the nine essential amino acids.

Kale

Edamame

Collard greens

Quinoa

Spinach

Beans

Nuts

Soy

Tofu

Broccoli

Soy milk

Almond milk

Hemp (protein powder)

Tempeh

Nut butter (peanut, almond, cashew)

Pumpkin seeds

Seitan

CARBOHYDRATES AND CARB SUBSTITUTES

1) ELIMINATE SUGAR First and foremost, you need to cut refined sugar from your diet. Nothing encourages greater release of insulin or contributes to increased fat more than consuming refined sugar in any form.

CUT OUT: Desserts, sugary sodas and sweet breakfast muffins. **Sugar is illegal in my playbook.**

2) ELIMINATE "STARCHY" CARBS. Greatly reduce other forms of carbs, even some you have been led to believe are healthy. The primary objective of my plan is to help you reduce bodyfat and position you to build muscle. Foods that you've been told are healthy may spike insulin release, which works against your current goal. This even includes whole grains, which you should only consume in moderation.

CUT OUT: Bread, pasta, rice (both brown and white), potatoes (white). If this is too much to ask at the beginning, then just reduce the amount and frequency of these foods you consume.

3) ELIMINATE SUGAR SUBSTITUTES. Drastically reduce or eliminate sugar substitutes such as aspartame (Equal, NutraSweet), sucralose (Splenda), saccharin (Sweet'N Low, SugarTwin), neotame, and acesulfame potassium (Sunett, Sweet One). These sugar substitutes are included in diet sodas and many other foods. Interestingly, these no-calorie molecules mimic the activity of sugar. So, even though they contain no calories, they do encourage the release of insulin. They negatively impact your ability to lose bodyfat nearly as much as refined sugars do. The only difference is that they don't include calories, but that doesn't matter, because these chemicals are encouraging your body to release insulin and drive other calories to fat storage.
CUT OUT: Diet sodas, desserts with sugar substitutes, and even "healthy" products that use these dietary sweeteners that cause insulin release.

4) CHECK INGREDIENT LABELS. Don't be fooled by sugar alcohols (strange name because they actually do not contain any alcohol at all). Sugar alcohols are carbohydrates that naturally occur in certain fruits and vegetables, but they can also be manufactured. They are lower in calories than regular sugars.

Sugar alcohols are generally found in many processed foods. The general public does not use them when cooking at home. Many protein bars that are low in carbs use sugar alcohols to help make the bars edible. If you find yourself with an upset stomach or bloating after eating certain processed foods, check to see if the product contains sugar alcohols. Many people have a problem digesting them and spend years trying to figure out why their stomach bloats and never gets flat.
CUT OUT: Sugar alcohols, which include erythritol, isomalt, lactitol, maltitol, mannitol, sorbitol and xylitol. Once you cut out sugar alcohols for about a week you may seem (and feel) far less bloating. Check ingredient labels.

5) EMPHASIZE FOODS HIGH IN FIBER. Interestingly, fiber is a form of carbohydrates that is indigestible. But that doesn't mean fiber is bad. In fact fiber plays a crucial role in mitigating blood sugar and insulin release. Fiber does this by slowing absorption of other calories, causing less insulin release. And fiber also prevents some calories from entering your body, sweeping them through. This is a benefit because fiber makes you feel fuller while helping you consume fewer calories.

There are two types of fiber: soluble and insoluble. Soluble fiber dissolves in water, and it is known to help decrease blood cholesterol, slow digestion, and delay intestinal absorption of sugar and starch. As a result, soluble fiber helps keep insulin spikes lower.

Insoluble fiber is known for both regulating and speeding up digestion. Insoluble fiber also bulks up your stool, so if you are constipated this type of fiber is crucial. You can't have ripped abs if you're always constipated and bloated, so being regular is crucial to you achieving six-pack abs and reduced bodyfat. Consuming fiber is a good way to accomplish this.

ADD IN: Most high-fiber foods have both soluble and insoluble fiber, but some foods have more of one than the other. Oats, fresh fruit, and some vegetables are very high in soluble fiber. The average person should strive to consume between 20-35 g of fiber per day, combining both types of fiber.

FOOD HIGH IN SOLUBLE FIBER

Bran

Barley

Nuts

Seeds

Beans

Lentils

Peas

Avocado

Brussels sprouts

Broccoli

Asparagus

Apples

Pears

Oranges

Figs

Dates

FOODS HIGH IN INSOLUBLE FIBER

Wheat

Bran

Whole-grain foods

Most vegetables

Turnips

Okra

Green peas

Asparagus

Beets

Sweet potato

Broccoli

Brussels sprouts

Corn

Kale

Green beans

All berries

Apples

Apricots

Figs

Oranges

Pears

Plums

Net Carbs

Many people get confused when they see a label that says "net carbs," and a number associated with it. What that means is the total number of grams of carbs in a food minus the total amount of grams of fiber in that food. That's because fiber is not absorbed, so it contains no calories. Consuming fiber will never by itself raise your insulin levels or spike your blood sugar. The more fiber a food has, the lower on the glycemic load list it tends to be (I'll explain glycemic load later). Fiber has great health and fat-loss benefits.

DIETARY FAT SOURCES

I haven't discussed dietary fats, yet, but I'm going to say something that may surprise you: You shouldn't fear dietary fats when you're on a fat-loss program. In fact, you need to eat fats to lose fat. Why is that? Because dietary fats don't spike insulin levels nearly as much as carbs and protein. Yes, even protein encourages the release of insulin.

If you include three of the foods from any of the "healthy fat foods" list, then you'll be consuming the fats you need to provide the proper amount of calories with the satiety you need to reduce bodyfat. While you should emphasize healthy fats (especially omega-3s), you shouldn't fear saturated fats. These are the fats that naturally occur in meats and dairy products.

On the other hand, there is one source of fats you should avoid as much (or more) than sugar. These are trans fats. These are chemically altered fats that have been proved to cause myriad health problems. In fact, trans fats are the reason saturated fats got their bad rap in the first place. Virtually every diet and informed nutritionist excludes trans fats from their recommendations because of how harmful they are.

First, though, let's start with the healthy fats:

HEALTHY FAT FOODS

While many of these foods are high in protein, they should also be the foods you rely on to get many of your fats. Lean meats contain a proper amount of saturated fats that will help you succeed on your diets. Avocados, nuts and seeds contain healthy omega fats that support long-term health, satiety and weight loss when consumed in moderation.

Lean beef
Chicken
Turkey
Pork
Whole eggs
Avocado
Nuts
Flax seeds

HEALTHY OILS

These foods contain a much higher amount of fats by percentage—some oils are 100% dietary fats, constituted of varying ratios of saturated and unsaturated fats. The more saturated fats the oil contains, then generally the cloudier or more solid it becomes with refrigeration.

MCT oil
Olive
Macadamia
Canola
Peanut
Soybean
Sunflower
Safflower

HEALTHY FATTY FISH

Fish is both an excellent source of protein and dietary fats. While some types of fish are very lean, the following fish contain a high amount of healthy fats, which are otherwise consumed in too low of a quantity in most people's diets.

Salmon
Mackerel
Rainbow trout
Bluefin tuna
Yellowfin tuna
Arctic char
Albacore
Skipjack tuna
Black cod
Chilean sea bass
Sardines

HEALTHY FATS BUT NOT PREFERRED (EAT SPARINGLY)

These foods are higher in dietary fats than those you should consume on a fat-loss program. Still, you can include them infrequently and in small portions. Just make sure to follow the portion adjustments I recommend later in the book.

Fattier beef
Lamb
Duck
Coconut oil
Full-fat cheese
Butter
Ghee
Lard
Goose fat

TRANS FATS FOODS

Look for the ingredient "partially hydrogenated oil" on nutrition panels and avoid these foods, entirely.

Margarine
Doughnuts
Fried anything
Frozen pizza
Cream-filled candies
Frosting
Biscuits
Breakfast sandwiches
Microwave Popcorn (opt for ones with labels that read "trans-fat free")

YOUR ACTION PLAN

▶ Cut out all refined sugar (and sugar substitutes)
▶ Reduce other carbs sources (especially starchy sources)
▶ Emphasize quality "primary proteins"
▶ Don't fear dietary fat; include it in moderation so long as you avoid trans fats

RULE #4:
FOLLOW THE GLYCEMIC LOAD PRINCIPLE

Every food affects insulin response in a unique way. Many years ago, scientists tested most foods to determine their impact on insulin release, which led to the development of the glycemic index. The glycemic index rates foods from 0-100 on how much the food raises your blood sugar levels.

This seems perfectly in keeping with what I've been preaching so far, doesn't it? But it's wrong, and the answer is to look at glycemic load rather than the glycemic index. Let me guide you through both of these.

FLAWS IN THE GLYCEMIC INDEX

The glycemic index is based on how much each food encourages insulin release when you eat it alone and in large quantities. No one eats a meal that has only one food. It indicates how quickly a specific food is digested and released as glucose (sugar) into your blood stream.

Foods with a high glycemic index raise your blood sugar more than those with a low glycemic index rating. The way they tested this was by having subjects consume an amount of every food that contains 50 g of carbohydrates, and then they tested blood sugar levels. But they neglected to tell you that 50 g of carbs from different foods vary fairly significantly from the amount you'd normally consume.

For instance, if you're going to consume 50 g of carbs from watermelon, you're going to have to take in about 60 oz or five cups of this fruit! And watermelon scores a 72 on the glycemic index scale, an undesirable number. But the glycemic load for watermelon is 7.2, making it acceptable on my nutrition plan. Based on the glycemic index alone, you would never eat watermelon because you'd believe that it would spike insulin release and cause you to store these calories as fat. But you're not going to eat an entire watermelon—and nothing else—for your dinner. Are you?

The better way to view how foods impact insulin release is through their glycemic load, which takes into account how much of a food you consume in a typical serving, as well as how you should mix them together. That's why I base my food recommendations on glycemic load.

THE GLYCEMIC LOAD PRINCIPLE

The answer is to look at glycemic load, a scale developed by nutrition scientists at Harvard that takes your portions of each food into account, rather than the glycemic index, which compares unrealistic quantities of individual foods based on their carbohydrate content. The difference is crucial. In addition, you can further reduce insulin release by pairing foods together. I'm going to address that in more detail in Chapter 5, but it's an important point to mention now, before I go into it in more depth later.

SCORING FOODS ON THE GLYCEMIC LOAD PRINCIPLE

The glycemic load is a ranking system for carbohydrate foods, and the scale runs from 0-60. This measures the amount of carbohydrates and the impact of each food from one typical serving. Foods that are in the 0-10-range are considered low; those in the 11-20-range rank as moderate, and those above 20 are high and should be eaten sparingly. Here's how it works.

Take for example watermelon. Watermelon is very high on the glycemic index, rating a 72. But on the glycemic load scale it is quite low, coming in at 7.2 based on the fact that the typical serving is one cup (8 oz). This amount of watermelon doesn't have many carbohydrates. It's mostly water.

Carrots are another low glycemic-load food that scores high on the glycemic index (71), but low in its glycemic load score (6).

In my food plan, you'll emphasize foods with a low glycemic load. I'll get into this in more detail in Chapter 5 where I explain how to pair foods together, which will broaden your food choices. Then I'll provide you with recipes that take glycemic load and insulin release into account.

YOUR ACTION PLAN

▶ Take the glycemic load of foods into account
▶ Know that the glycemic index is flawed based on unfair quantity comparisons
▶ Read Chapter 5 to better understand how to construct your diet based on the much more accurate glycemic load

RULE #5:
GET YOUR PORTIONS RIGHT

In terms of portion control, this is literally in your hands. Your hand will become your calorie monitor without you ever having to count a calorie. For any given meal, you must first decide which source of protein you'll be eating. Then you'll determine your carbohydrate source per meal.

If your goal is to reduce bodyfat and weight, then you should limit your protein portion to approximately the size of your palm, which includes the heel of your hand and first row of knuckles (length and thickness). If you want to maintain your current weight and just drop fat, limit your protein portion to the size of your entire hand. If you would like to gain a lot of muscle and increase total bodyweight, then your protein portion should be the size of your entire hand plus a half of your other hand.

On the other hand, if you only eat two meals a day, then your protein can

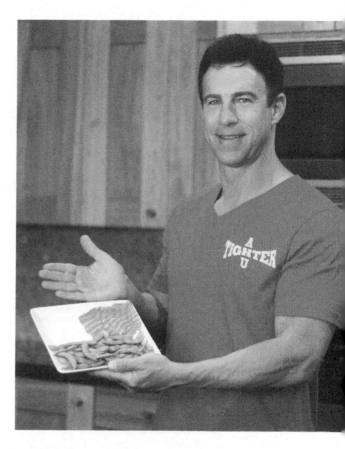

A meal of salmon sashimi and edamame is my favorite lunch. I often eat it 2-3 times a week. You can vary your foods as much as you want. The size of the protein here is palm and first row of knuckles.

start as your entire hand instead of your first row of knuckles. If you want to maintain your current weight, your protein can be the size of your whole hand plus a half, and if you want to gain large amounts of muscle then go with then two full hands for each meal.

HAND-SIZE PORTIONS

These three diagrams provide examples of how you should measure your protein serving for each meal. For more diagrams and insight on using hand portions, go to **atighteru.com**.

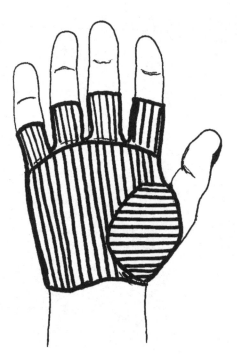

Reduce both bodyfat and weight

When this is your goal, limit your protein for each meal to a portion size equal to your palm plus the heel of your hand and first row of knuckles.

Carb Portions

⭐ Based on your choice of protein, you will determine which carbohydrates you should appropriately pair with that protein and the quantity of each. I'll give you more details about this in Chapter 5, where I provide you with the scores for carbohydrates on the glycemic load scale.

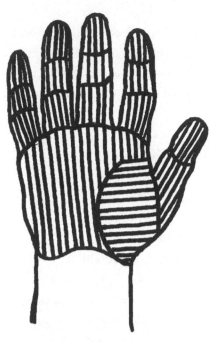

Maintain your weight and lose bodyfat

When this is your goal, consume a piece of primary protein that's equal to the size of your full hand.

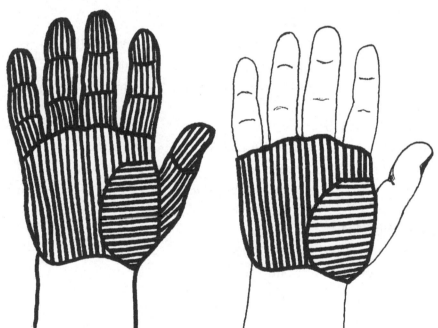

Gain muscle and lose bodyfat

When this is your goal, you should consume a protein serving that's equal to the size of your full hand plus half of your other hand.

Suffice it to say for now that if you choose a carb food that is low on the glycemic load scale, then you can eat about double the amount as compared to what you're consuming for protein, but if you choose a carb with higher glycemic load, then you should eat about an equal volume of carbs as compared to your protein portion.

I call this the 1:2 or the 1:1.5 or 1:1 ratio. Here's how it works;

If you choose a good protein =1, then:
You choose a low GL carb = 2 (double size of carbs to protein, and you can have more than one type of these carbs)
You choose a medium GL carb = 1.5   (1.5 size carb as protein)
You choose a GL high carb = 1 (same size carb serving as protein)
Here are quick examples of each of these carb options after you choose a quality protein source. You can also see photos demonstrating this concept on page 88-91.

EXAMPLE: 1:2 RATIO

PROTEIN	LOW CARB	LOW CARB
Chicken breast	Broccoli	Cauliflower
	(same size as protein)	(same size as protein)

EXAMPLE 1:1.5

PROTEIN	MEDIUM CARB	MEDIUM CARB
Chicken breast	Lentils	Sweet potato
	(3/4 size of the protein)	(3/4 size of the protein)

EXAMPLE 1:1

PROTEIN	HIGH CARB
Chicken breast	Risotto
	(same size as the protein)

YOUR ACTION PLAN

▶ Choose your protein portion based on your physique goal
▶ Select a carb source that balances your protein portion and allows for satiety
▶ Read Chapter 5 to better understand how to pair foods together

RULE #6:
TAKE BCAAS BEFORE AND AFTER YOUR WORKOUTS

I believe that you should get most of your nutrients from food. One exception is branched-chain amino acids (BCAAs). BCAAs are a group of three essential amino acids: leucine, isoleucine and valine. They're the basics of protein molecules, which means they are a macronutrient. Yet BCAAs are unique and should be supplemented because we don't get in enough from our food supply.

BCAAs are essential amino acids. The term "essential" means something different here than it typically does. In the context of amino acids, the "essential" ones are those that your body cannot make from other amino acids, making it necessary to get them through your food or supplements. Essential amino acids often provide specific advantages, but they are not typically as necessary for survival or crucial physiological functions. Our bodies have become expert chemists when it comes to making non-essential amino acids. These are the ones we need most for health and survival. Yeah, I know, the names feel a little off, but these are the scientific terms for them.

BCAAs are very crucial "essential amino acids," providing unique advantages. In particular, BCAAs promote muscle protein synthesis and, therefore, muscle growth. Research also suggests that BCAAs provide additional muscular energy during workouts, allowing you to perform more reps in a set.

WHY BCAAS WORK

BCAAs are a crucial part of my program. They not only promote muscle growth, but they also encourage your body to burn fat. The more muscle a person has, the more calories they burn daily to sustain the muscle they have.

The key is to get your body to preferentially burn fat. Remember that one of the biggest reasons diets fail is that people lose muscle mass, which makes it more challenging to burn bodyfat. Supplementing BCAAs when you're on a fat-loss program will help you maintain muscle mass while improving your body's ability to burn stored fat.

BCAAs encourage your body to release insulin to achieve their advantages. This may sound like something you don't want (unless you read my chapter on insulin very carefully). But you actually want your body to release insulin immediately after your workouts. And, depending on your goal and workout, it may be desirable to release insulin before you train.

HOW BCAAS WORK

BCAAs are not synthesized in your liver (where amino acids are converted to carbs), so they are transported throughout your body as amino acids. Insulin transports BCAAs directly to working muscle tissue to help repair the damage your workouts cause. This encourages muscle growth and faster recovery, providing you with more energy the next time you workout. This won't make you bulkier, because more muscle fibers fit into a small space.

Muscle fibers are lined with insulin receptors, like a dock for a boat. Once the insulin docks, it tells the muscle cell to allow glucose and amino acids to enter the muscle. This docking increases protein synthesis, which is fundamental for building muscle and speeding recovery.

Once your body uses the glucose in the muscles and liver to fuel the workout—which won't last all that long—it then calls on the stored energy in your fat cells to continue to power your workout. Now you're cutting directly into your stored fat to fuel your training! That is the key part to the benefits of my workouts and my program.

HOW TO TAKE BCAAS

Many people recommend that you take BCAAs with other supplements and ingredients, such as protein shakes that are high in sugar or sugar substitutes. But these other calories often end up preventing fat from being released to fuel your workouts or getting stored in fat cells. So, you should take BCAAs with water or other low- or no-calorie beverages, such as black coffee or tea.

My program is based on timing. It is essential you take your BCAAs within five minutes of starting your weightlifting and right after you finish. If you are doing your cardio right after, take your BCAAs when you finish your cardio.

On days when you split your cardio and weights, take the BCAAs before and after your workouts. Do the same thing on days when you just do cardio. BCAAs are still beneficial for supporting recovery from cardio because that type of training also breaks down muscle tissue.

BCAAs will slightly spike your insulin levels for a very short period and drive the amino acids straight into your muscles.

People might say, "Wait a minute. If you're spiking your insulin won't this shut off your fat burning? Shouldn't I take BCAAs only after (but not before) my weight-training workouts?"

Pure BCAAs stimulate a quick insulin response after taking them. Since there are no carbohydrates in your system at this time (if you're following my program), then your insulin spike will be very short. The amino acids are delivered right into the muscle to keep them from breaking down and fuel immediate exercise. The short interruption in fat burning is well worth it because instead of losing muscle, you're setting up your body to build muscle and lose more bodyfat over time.

Immediately after your weightlifting session take your second dose of BCAAs and eat a meal if the timing is right. A great time for a meal is directly after a weight-lifting session, but this is a challenge unless you're training 4-5 hours after your previous meal. If your schedule doesn't allow for a meal right after your workout, then at least take your BCAAs. That will start your muscle recovery and building process, which will boost your metabolism for more effective fat burning.

MORE MUSCLE, BETTER METABOLISM

While some people like to take in some form of artificial metabolism booster, all you're really getting is caffeine or some other form of natural speed. The problem with these products is they only last for a short time. The best way to up your metabolism to boost fat loss is to add lean muscle. And muscle mass is the best and cheapest fat-burner out there. Building muscle is the name of the game when it comes to upping your metabolism, and with the right supplementation at the right time you can build it easily.

I train models, actors/actresses, professional and Olympic athletes, and bodybuilders. The one thing they all have in common besides having me as their trainer is that I have all of them taking BCAAs. My preference is BCAAs from Hollywood Supps.

YOUR ACTION PLAN

▸ BCAAs boost metabolism, build muscle and help reduce stored fat
▸ Take at least 3 g of BCAAs five minutes before your weight-training workouts
▸ Take at least 3 g of BCAAs immediately after your full workout

RULE #7:
DRINK THE RIGHT FLUIDS

One of the primary rules of every fat-loss program is that you need to watch the beverages you consume. That's true on mine as well. Beverages full of calories provide very little satiety, and they often cause a spike in insulin. This won't surprise you: You'll be cutting out beverages that spike insulin.

But you should also up your fluid-intake game when you're on a fat-loss program. Remember I said earlier that one of the problems with most diets is that you lose water weight, but you don't lose fat? Well, you don't want to lose water weight. That means you need to stay well hydrated.

Here are my rules-within-a-rule:

1) Avoid fruit juices.

You may have been told a glass of orange juice in the morning is one of the healthiest things you can consume. No piece of nutritional advice could be more wrong. Fruit juice is one of the worst things you can take in when you're trying to reduce bodyfat. Pure fruit juice contains nothing but carbohydrates (sugar) with virtually zero fiber. Drinking it drives insulin release through the roof! One glass of orange juice contains the fruit from multiple oranges (between 5-7), but without the beneficial fiber that whole oranges contain. In addition, fruit juice is very high in fructose, a type of sugar you particularly want to avoid.

On the other hand, it's perfectly fine to consume whole fruits that are high in fiber such as oranges, papayas, pineapples or grapefruits. That's because the fiber in these fruits reduces the release of insulin, making them acceptable food choices on my fat-loss program. In addition, these foods have a low glycemic load due to their low amount of calories per serving.

2) Avoid other sugary and sugar-substitute beverages.

You already know that sugar causes an unwanted release of insulin. Sugary sodas (and other beverages) often contain high-fructose corn syrup, or other ridiculously unhealthy versions. This type of sugar is even more damaging to your health and fat-loss program than table sugar (sucrose). Even companies such as Coke and Pepsi have started marketing new versions of their sugary beverages, touting that they contain sucrose, which is less harmful than high-fructose corn syrup.

And, as I explained earlier, even diet sweeteners trigger the release of insulin.

Again, that's because these chemicals mimic the structure of "real" sugars, and your body responds in kind, releasing insulin, which you don't want most times of day.

3) Avoid "healthy" caloric beverages.

Even vegetable beverages are suspect. Once again, these remove the fiber in favor of "nutrients." But these nutrients take a backseat to the damage that vegetable juice causes due its sugar content and subsequent insulin release. Keep in mind that even protein shakes cause an insulin release. You can take these in after workouts to provide amino acids, but these products cause your body to release insulin, which spikes appetite. And that's not what you're seeking on a fat-loss program. Sure, protein shakes can be beneficial if you're trying to add muscle mass and bodyweight, but be careful about how you consume them when you're trying to shed bodyfat.

You should avoid "healthy" sports beverages. You've seen commercials that show athletes downing them during a game to give themselves an extra boost. One look at the labels and you can see that they're full of sugar, and they're going to spike insulin release. These products will support activity, but they do so in addition to causing insulin release, which you need to avoid in order to lose fat.

4) Consume at least two liters of water a day.

Many times we feel hungry when we're actually thirsty. Most people do not drink enough water, and they find themselves eating food instead of just downing a glass of water, which is what their body is actually seeking. While food contains water, it's a huge waste of calories to consume food when your body is thirsting for water. In general, if you're having a craving, I recommend that you consume a glass of water before you give in to any temptation.

Water provides many other health benefits, as well. It flushes out your kidneys and digestive system, hydrating your body and brain, allowing your metabolism to function more effectively. You also look healthier when you're well hydrated.

5) Drink water, tea, and coffee.

Coffee and tea are both loaded with antioxidants, and they're mostly water. In addition they are virtually calorie free. You can drink these beverages hot or cold, but don't add sugars or sugar substitutes, or consume diet drinks, which cause unwanted insulin spikes.

While you should consume two liters of water a day on its own, you can also think of your coffee and tea drinks contributing to your water consumption. Many people argue that coffee and tea are "dehydrating," but that's ultimately not true. If you ate tea leaves or coffee beans, perhaps you'd be less hydrated, but consuming these beverages with water makes this a nonsensical point. Still, strive to get in two liters of water, however much coffee or tea you drink. The fluid in coffee and tea are a bonus.

6) Drink raw, unfiltered apple cider vinegar diluted in water before every meal. Recent studies suggest that drinking two tablespoons of raw, unfiltered apple cider vinegar diluted in 12 oz of water may have significant health benefits. It lowers blood pressure and acid reflux, and it supports weight loss and the health of diabetics. You can probably guess the reason for the latter: it reduces insulin spikes.

A study performed at Arizona State University concluded that drinking apple cider vinegar before meals and at bedtime reduced post-meal and fasting glucose levels by up to 40%. By drinking this mixture right before you start to eat, not 20 minutes before but right before, you return to the Burn Zone much more quickly.

People who regularly consume this apple cider vinegar beverage have reported feeling more full between meals, although that has not been scientifically proved. But this makes sense to me—reducing insulin release helps decrease appetite. This can put you in the Burn Zone for about 1.5 more hours per day, because it reduces insulin release by about 30%.

I've stressed the importance of keeping insulin levels low with the shortest spikes possible. Including watered-down, raw, unfiltered apple cider vinegar is an essential component of my fat-loss program. *Do not* drink it straight because it can lead to an upset stomach and irritate your throat; always dilute it with water. By drinking it unfiltered, you can add up to 1.5 hours of the Burn Zone to your day. I even add a little lemon or lime to reduce the taste of vinegar. Lately, I've been adding sparkling water with no calories or diet sweeteners, also a good option.

YOUR ACTION PLAN

- ▶ Drink at least 2 liters of water every day
- ▶ Avoid fruit juices and other sugary beverages, including sodas and sports drinks
- ▶ Consume raw apple cider vinegar diluted with water before every meal
- ▶ Drink coffee and tea without added calories as you want

RULE #8:
FOLLOW THE RULES, BUT ALLOW YOURSELF A CHEAT MEAL

By now you should know that you can't have a rule without an exception and so here is mine: Once a week you should consume a cheat meal, consuming whatever you want.

It's important that you still follow all of the other rules at every other meal throughout the week, but a cheat meal provides benefits. In fact, you're not—exactly—cheating; rather, you're supporting your fat-loss program.

When you're on a disciplined program, your body accommodates to the amount of calories you consume, regardless of how much you're controlling insulin release. I mentioned earlier that taking in food causes your body to rev up its fat burning. Of course it doesn't do that to the extent that it burns all of the calories you're consuming. But digestion does burn calories. Taking in a cheat meal once a week encourages your body to rev up metabolism to digest this unexpected intake of food. But when you do this frequently (especially every day), your body gets used to this huge influx of calories, and it just expects them and stores them as bodyfat.

Cheating once a week also sends your body the signal that it's not in starvation mode, and it doesn't need to hoard bodyfat.

Here are my guidelines for cheat meals:

Plan your cheat meal in advance. Make this meal as important as every other meal. You can eat whatever you want in this meal, but it's good to include protein, fats, and fiber. You can also add some refined sugar. This once-a-week insulin spike will not ruin your diet; in fact, it may better support it.

Keep calorie intake moderately high: It's a cheat meal—you can go a little nuts. You can take in 1,000-1,500 calories during this meal, depending on your bodyweight and muscle content. For example, one slice of cheese pizza has about 285 calories. The more muscle you have, the more calories you can consume during the meal. Just don't turn it into a full-out gorge fest.

Contain your cheat window. One of the best ways to prevent yourself from "over cheating" is to keep your "cheat meal" window to about two hours. Don't cheat before, and don't cheat afterwards. It's not a free-for-all.

- ▶ Cheat only for one meal once a week
- ▶ Plan your cheat meal and eat whatever foods you want
- ▶ Keep quantities to no more than "moderately large"
- ▶ Contain your cheat window to 2 hours

RULE #9:
SLEEP LONG AND DEEP

According to the Center for Disease Control and Prevention, more than 35% of Americans are sleep deprived. What's intriguing is that the statistics for obesity are nearly identical. I'm not suggesting that every person who doesn't get enough sleep is obese, but I am suggesting there's likely a link between the two.

Getting in less than seven hours of sleep per night, especially over extended periods, has many deleterious effects. It's no shock that lack of sleep undoes or diminishes your weight-loss goals. Who wants to train when they're tired? You may not want to go to bed, but you'll be more likely to go home and sit on the couch for an extra hour rather than head to the gym if you're under-rested.

Research also suggests that getting too little sleep negatively impacts the effects of insulin. Studies show that four consecutive nights of poor sleep reduces a person's insulin sensitivity by up to 30%. That means that your body will need to release more insulin even though you're not consuming excess calories, and those calories will more likely be driven to fat storage.

When you sleep long and deep, your body also releases several important hormones, including growth factors such as IGF-I, which support muscle-building, recovery from training, and ultimately fat-loss. This alone could explain why under-sleeping fights against your fat-loss goals.

In addition, lack of sleep also stimulates appetite even though you're not burning that many more calories by being awake.

Some good news about my plan, and how it supports sleep: Because you'll be eating no more than three meals per day, you'll be unlikely to be digesting food into the night, which also disrupts sleep.

Here are my eight tips on how to get a better night's sleep.

GET YOUR ZZZS

1) Take melatonin.

Melatonin is a hormone found in the human body. Melatonin helps regulate the sleep and waking cycle, and it helps balance your hormones. In addition, the human body releases growth hormone and reduces cortisol secretion during sleep. The deeper and longer you sleep the better your body will work the next day.

Ingesting supplemental melatonin may help you sleep better, lose body-fat, gain muscle mass and function more effectively. I use Hollywood Supps Melatonin to provide an extra boost of this critical hormone. The best time to take it is just as you're getting into bed. This version of melatonin is delivered as a gummy, which is better than a pill or liquid because the gummy acts as a transport system, delivering the melatonin more efficiently. Since the total calorie count of each dose is under 10, the gummy will not spike your insulin levels.

Keep in mind that as a person ages, the natural level of melatonin production decreases. That makes melatonin supplementation more important as you get older to support better health.

2) Drink plenty of water throughout the day.

Dehydration causes your heart rate to increase even during sleep. Going to bed hydrated helps you sleep longer, better and deeper. Consider drinking water if you awake during the night unless you know that will further disrupt sleep due to a need to use the bathroom.

3) Go to bed at the same time every night.

And get up at the same time every morning to create a natural sleep rhythm. The more regular your sleep patterns, the better advantages you'll gain from sleep, and from my program in general, as it will help you better plan your full 24-hour cycle with meals and workouts.

4) Avoid alcohol.

Alcohol is not only unhealthy, but it disrupts your sleep patterns. While many people use alcohol to help them get to sleep, it often disrupts sleep later in the cycle (or prevents you from getting into deeper more restful stages of sleep). When good sleep and fat loss are your goals, avoid alcohol.

5) Hide your clock

Set your alarm, but don't watch the clock when you wake up in the middle of the night. It's easy enough to do — set your clock within reach, but turn the face so that you can't see it when you're lying down.

6) Wear socks to bed.

A Swiss study published in *Nature* observed warm hands and feet are the fastest way to fall asleep. https://www.nature.com/articles/43366

7) Perform self-acupressure.

Between your eyebrows and above your nose is a pressure point. Apply gentle pressure for 1 minute. Breathe in and out slowly as you do this to help slow your heart rate and relax yourself.

8) Shut off the TV and put on classical music.

It will either lull you to sleep or bore you to the point where sleep will be the best escape. Keep the volume low, and set a timer to turn it off, if possible.

YOUR ACTION PLAN

▶ Sleep is an important part of good health
▶ It's also crucial for supporting fat loss
▶ Follow the tips in this section for better sleep

RULE #10:
KEEP TRACK OF YOUR FAT-LOSS RESULTS

Those before-and-after photos exist for a reason: They're extremely effective at marketing any fat-loss or muscle-building nutrition or training program. That's a bit psychological, a way to entice you to buy into a certain program, and spend money on everything they're selling.

But that's not the only reason for those shots: They're also hyper-motivating for those on the program. You get frequent feedback, and you're able to see your improvements in a variety of ways. While many of these "quick-fix" programs are bogus, they rely on actual motivators. My program delivers long-term fat-loss, and I want you to use these metrics to keep track of your progress over the long haul.

I strongly suggest you keep track of your changes from the start of your program through the finish line. These aren't marketing and hype when they're *your* results. They're real. And they're really motivating.

That's the topic of the next chapter.

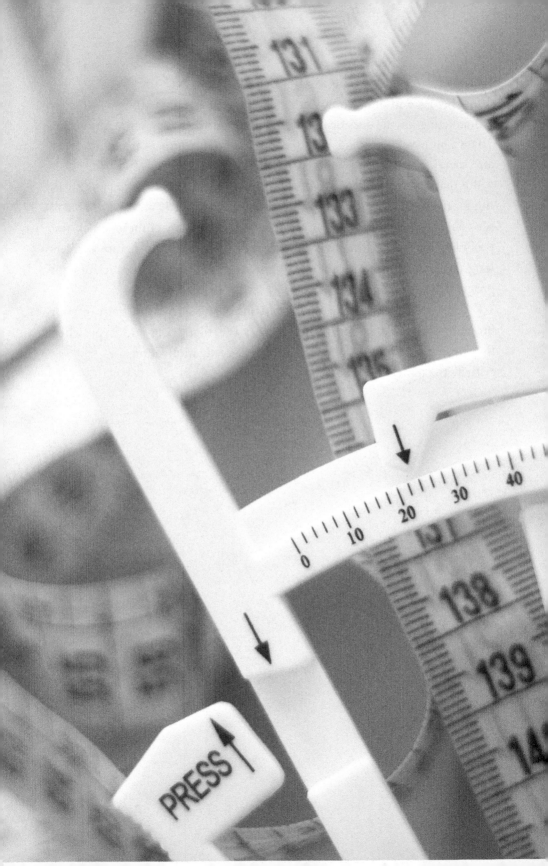

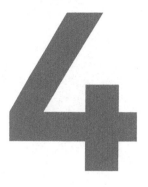

CHAPTER

4

GETTING STARTED

Use Your Scale Wisely

Keep one thing in mind: bodyweight can be deceptive. Looking—and feeling—great is not about the number on your scale.

When you're following my program, you engage in both weightlifting and aerobic exercise. You will increase muscle density, but not necessarily muscle size, unless you lift weights in a way designed to build muscle mass. Some female clients worry about getting too big, but I promise you that just does not happen. One pound of muscle takes up about half the space compared to a pound of fat. So, it is entirely possible for your bodyweight to increase after gaining muscle, while your waist size decreases significantly.

Don't freak out if your bodyweight increases. Don't worry about the number on your scale. The goal is to change your body, not a number. The tools to chart your progress are a mirror and how your clothes fit. And, of course, how you feel.

In collaboration with BuzzFeed, I shot a video called "We lost 22% of Bodyfat in 6 Weeks." (https://youtu.be/TNQ8ZKq9QQ0). During this process, producer Ashley Perez gained 4 pounds on the scale but she dropped two dress sizes in six weeks, and went from 24% bodyfat down to 18%. That means she lost 25% of her bodyfat! That's a huge change.

She began at 136 pounds and ended at 140 pounds. But in the process she dropped 8 pounds of fat. Ashley told me this is the best she has ever looked, and now she's incredibly comfortable in her own skin.

That's the goal.

Think of your muscles as a 12-cylinder gas guzzling Ferrari—the more muscle fibers you have, the more calories your body will burn every day, even at rest. If you have a small amount of muscle fibers then your body will function more like a moped—performing more with far less fuel. A moped person can eat the same thing as a Ferrari person, but they will end up storing the excess as fat for later use because they lack the muscle to burn it off.

SUPERHERO STORY:
Reboot Your Body

⭐ Zach Dresler trained with me for six weeks for the "We Lost 22% of Bodyfat in 6 Weeks" video, and he lost 30.1 pounds of bodyfat. Of course, he also added muscle mass.

"Steve Zim taught me what I need to eat and how to train," Zach says. "It was a hard-line crash course, but he rebooted my body."

While we finished up our six-week program a couple years ago, Zach still trains at my gym in Culver City.

"Sometimes I ask Steve for tips on form or questions about nutrition, but he taught me how to take charge of my own program." Zach keeps his nutrition clean to this day. "I add in a cheat meal one day a week or so because now that I have my engine going, I can maintain the fat loss and have a few more cheat meals here and there."

Zach adds a word of encouragement for others who are just starting out: "It may sound overwhelming at first, but when you simplify Steve's program and follow it consistently for 2-3 months, you'll not only improve the way you look, but you'll increase your chances for a longer life."

Thinking of yourself as a top-of-the-line Ferrari is a confidence builder. Millions of people spend hours every year buying self-help books and finding ways to achieve happiness. Gaining the physical self-confidence that Ashley achieved in six weeks can go a long way to improving all areas of your life. If you don't love your body, achieving other goals that make you happy are more difficult. Let's fix it together.

Here's what you need to get started.

PUT YOUR SCALE IN PERSPECTIVE

Because weight loss and weight gain are emotionally charged issues for many people, it's important that you don't get hung up on bodyweight numbers. Your actual weight can be deceptive. Keep in mind that the number on the scale to measure "progress " must be redefined.

First of all… let's be realistic. Do you truly care how much you weigh on a scale or would you rather be the same size you were when you were happiest with your body? Have you spent your whole life trying to get to the point where you say, "Sure I'll put on a bathing suit and go to the beach with my friends?" If you were five pounds heavier than you are today but were three sizes smaller, would you complain?

Unless you have to make weight for a boxing or wrestling match, body-weight alone is irrelevant. Bodyweight is only one aspect of four that tells the full story of what is going on with your body:

1) Scale and bodyweight
2) Physical measurements (hips, waist, etc.)
3) Bodyfat test
4) Before and after photos

By keeping track of these four distinct metrics, you get a much clearer picture of what is happening in your body. It's how you know if you're changing in the right way. These measurements are available and accessible to everyone and can accurately determine the amount of muscle, bone density, and fat you gain and lose. Let me go through each of them:

BODYWEIGHT

When you step onto a scale, you are weighing muscle, fat and other important bodyparts, including water, hair, organs and bone. But clearly, you shouldn't care how much your hair, organs and bones weigh. These, essentially, aren't things you can change to improve your health and appearance.

When you rely only on your scale it's much harder to maintain your new set point than it is to reach it. When most people lose a large amount of scale weight, they also lose much needed muscle mass and water. They reduce the power of the engine that burns the fat. And the greater the loss of muscle tissue, the harder it is for you to maintain weight loss over the long term. So don't use scale weight, especially alone, as a measure of your success.

BODYPART MEASUREMENTS

Take your measurements before you begin your nutrition program. When you have your measurements taken, it is important to do so prior to exercise. Don't take them after you lift or do cardio because they won't be accurate. Knowing your measurements is crucial for several reasons.

First, accurate measurements give you a sense of your body's symmetry. As your body transforms over the course of the program, these initial measurements help to determine which parts of your body need more or less work.

For instance, some of my male clients often notice a sudden appearance of love handles upon progressing through my program. So, what is going on? Using a tape measure, I show them they actually lost a few inches around their waist, but many more inches around their trunk. In one specific case, upon measuring the area surrounding the belly button, my client had lost three inches despite his newly visible "love handles."

We can't choose from which part of our bodies we shed fat first. Our bodies do that for us. Muscle, on the other hand, can be gained or lost in targeted areas of the body depending on your exercise regimen, but that's a more detailed discussion for my next book. For every person, there are areas that shed fat more easily than others. Once you've burned fat from those easier areas, your body will intuitively begin targeting the fat located in the more reluctant areas. At that point, your progress will be apparent on a near daily basis.

BODYFAT PERCENTAGE

Measuring your bodyfat percentage is an essential step in assessing your physical status, both when you start and to track your progress. There are a variety of methods used to perform this measurement, ranging in price from free to $15 to $15,000. The most accurate bodyfat test is the water submersion test, but if it's not readily available and affordable, then many gyms have a skinfold or scale bodyfat test available, or else they can refer you to someone who can perform this test.

Calipers typically measure the fat content beneath the skin from three to five different parts of your body. Then, using both your scale weight and fat content, they calculate your bodyfat percentage. Often, you can have this measurement taken at the gym, by a licensed nutritionist, an accredited personal trainer, or by a general practitioner. This test can cost anywhere from $15 to $35 dollars, but its results are invaluable.

After this measurement is taken, you will know exactly how much of your total weight is comprised of fat, and how much is muscle. Instead of stepping on the scale every day to check your progress, have your bodyfat percentage measured every two weeks or so. Learning the ratios of fat to lean muscle mass is vital information that can truly change your perspective when addressing the sensitive topic of weight.

Bodyfat percentage standards differ by gender. An excellent bodyfat percentage for a man is 12% or somewhat lower, while for a woman it is 18% or somewhat lower. For reference, most competitive male athletes hover between 6-13% bodyfat; female athletes compete between 14-20 % bodyfat. Male bodybuilders compete at about 2-4 % on contest days, and female bodybuilders at about 4-6%.

It is VERY important to note that the moment a competition is over, bodybuilders resume their normal eating habits. By the next day, they will not look anything like they did on stage hours earlier. Many professional bodybuilders will gain twenty or more pounds during their off-season, enabling them to build more mass, from which they can later burn fat, resulting in an even larger percentage of lean muscle mass the next season. That's a bit of a tangent, but it's important, for realistic expectations, to know bodybuilders do not look competitively lean all of the time.

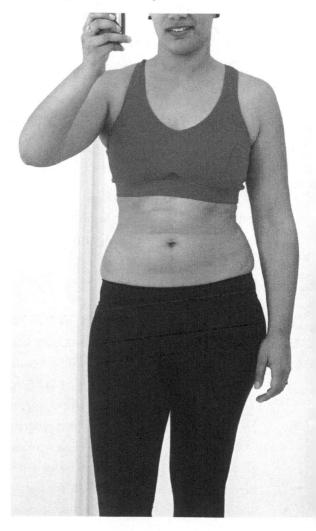

KEEP A VISUAL DIARY

On Day 1 take a front and back photo of yourself. Side photos are optional. Have a friend take the photos from about 10 feet away. Try to find a place where the light is even—in other words don't take a photo near a window or where there is a spotlight to one side. That can lead to a picture that makes you look uneven. One side could look flat while the other looks more cut.

For each pose, you should take two photos—one where you are relaxed and the other where you are flexing. This will allow you to see the changes in your appearance both ways—the posed one will help show increases in muscle mass as well as increased detail as you shed bodyfat.

SUPERHERO WORKOUT:
Hit the Books!

⭐ Working out with weights at least three days a week is essential to getting you to the Superhero body you're striving for. My next project is a fitness book titled Superhero Workout. But until that book comes out I'd like you to take a look at one of my previous books. I've already published three bestselling fitness books with workouts, and I believe they are still the best on the market today. What are out of date in these books are the nutrition and cardio sections, which is why I'm writing this book.

I recommend that you take pictures once a week—you don't want to do it too frequently because you won't see as much progress. But you don't want the interval to be too long either because you won't have as clear of a record of your fat loss.

Make sure you wear the same clothes every time and shoot the photos in the same place for a more accurate direct comparison.

I love using pictures to keep track of fat loss because they give you a great reality check, positive or negative. Pictures also help keep you highly motivated to continue your program.

You can find great workouts in my previously published books. These titles include:

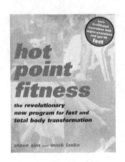

HOT POINT FITNESS
Publisher: De Capo Press Inc., 2000
My bestselling book, *Hot Point Fitness* is like having me training you at the gym. The book includes 3-, 4- and 5-day-a-week programs. This book also tells you how to choose which program is right for you. I include a progression for each workout for a full month to help you keep going. The book includes pictures and detailed descriptions of how to do all the exercises. This book is specifically for the gym — not home use. I believe this is one of the best fitness books ever written for the gym.

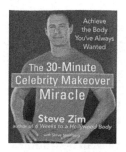

6 WEEKS TO A HOLLYWOOD BODY
Publisher: Wiley & Sons, 2006

This book is like having me train you at your home. You do not need to belong to a gym. This is a 3-day-a-week workout program that provides you with a regimen like those of the stars I train so that you can have a Hollywood body of your own. Unlike other books, this one provides programs based on your body type, whether you're an ectomorph, an endomorph, or a mesomorph — or a combination of two. I created specific training programs to suit each body type. I teach you how to figure out which type you are, and I give you the programs to follow.

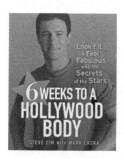

THE 30-MINUTE CELEBRITY MAKEOVER MIRACLE
Publisher: Wiley & Sons, 2007

This book is a 30-minute-a-day, three-times-a- week, combined cardio and weight-training program. It will help you ramp up your metabolic rate, burn fat faster than conventional workouts, and produce changes in your overall appearance. Every time you exercise you'll perform a different workout focused on balancing your body.

Cardio—Choose What Works for You

You should perform whatever type you like to do best. Here's a list of choices. You can perform these for 30-75 minutes per session. Keep in mind that including more intense sequences and then scaling back helps burn bodyfat more efficiently. Take a look at my more specific recommendations, based on your needs. First, here are some great types of cardio you can choose.

Running	Recumbent bike
Walking	Rowing
Jumping rope	Boxing
Stair climber	Hula-hoop
Elliptical	Swimming
Bike	And many others I have not listed.

MY CARDIO SUGGESTIONS

The best results and the least amount of injuries come from a modified interval program. Pick an amount of cardio that is right for you. If you're a beginner start slow. Beginners can walk 5 to 10 minutes to begin with; everyone needs to start somewhere. Your starting point is what it is, but what I'm more concerned with is where you are going.

If your bodyfat is where you want it to be, then do no more than 30 minutes of cardio four times a week. If you need to reduce bodyfat by 10% or more (from 32% to 22%, for example), then do no less than four days a week of a minimum of 30 minutes of cardio. Anyone needing to lose over 10% bodyfat or more should do at least five days of cardio for no less than 30 minutes a day. Everyone can do cardio if they like seven days a week but nobody should do more than 75 min of cardio a day.

Here is my cardio prescription for everyone once they feel ready and able to do at least 30 minutes of continuous walking. Go slow for one minute then sprint or go all out for 15-30 seconds. Repeat this interval for your allotted amount of cardio time. The idea is you are constantly driving your heart rate up then dropping it. In terms of weight loss, my intervals are more effective than long, slow endurance exercise, and they're also easier on your body long-term.

The intense effort you put in means that your body must work harder to recover, so you'll burn more calories in the 24 hours after an interval workout than you would after a slow, steady run. During those 24 hours after high-intensity interval training (known as HIIT), your body can also produce up to 450% more human growth hormone, which also increases caloric burn and supports muscle growth.

Studies have shown that interval cardio accelerates your heart rate, but actually decreases the strain on your heart. Over time, cardiovascular exercise can increase your heart stroke volume, or the amount of blood that your heart pumps per beat. Interval training maximizes cardiovascular benefits, so it can quickly increase stroke volume, making your heart stronger and more efficient.

I could go on and on, but the bottom line is it will get you leaner at 100 miles an hour faster than regular cardio.

KEEP TRACK OF YOUR PROGRESS

Whether you record your information in this book, download it from my website at www.atighteru.com or keep track of it somewhere else, these are the most important measurements and numbers you should keep track of to make certain your program is working. Record all of these before you start following my program, and then take them again each week before you workout.

MEASUREMENTS

	DATE	DATE	DATE	DATE	DATE	DATE	DATE
Bodyfat%	_____	_____	_____	_____	_____	_____	_____
Scale weight (pounds)	_____	_____	_____	_____	_____	_____	_____
Fat (pounds)	_____	_____	_____	_____	_____	_____	_____
Muscle	_____	_____	_____	_____	_____	_____	_____

Here's how you calculate your muscle mass, also known as lean body mass (which is composed of muscle, bone, tissue, water, and organs). It's everything except the fat below your skin.

Step 1) Subtract your bodyfat percentage from 100 to get your percent of lean mass

100 - Bodyfat % = Lean Mass %

Step 2) Turn that into a decimal by dividing by 100

$$\frac{\text{Lean Mass \%}}{100} = \text{Lean Mass \% as a decimal}$$

Step 3) Multiply your lean mass decimal by your total bodyweight to get your muscle mass in pounds

Lean Mass % decimal point x Total bodyweight = Lean Mass weight decimal point

Here is an example using a 200-lb person with 20% bodyfat:

100 - 20 = 80
80 / 100 = 0.80
0.80 x 200 = 160 (Lean Mass) and 40 pounds of bodyfat

Next, insert your measurements using a tape measure below. Make sure to take the measurements at the same place every time. Be sure to measure both sides.

DATE							
Neck							
Shoulders							
Chest							
Waist							
Hips							
	RT/LT	RT/LT	RT/LT	RT/LT	RT/LT	RT/LT	RT/LT
Thighs							
Calf							
Biceps							

Now let's take the information above one step further and figure out how many pounds of fat you have vs. how many pounds of lean body mass you have. This is very important because, as I told you earlier, many nutrition programs may make your bodyweight go down at the cost of losing lean muscle.

Remember, the goal of my program is to increase lean muscle, while decreasing bodyfat. If you decrease both, you will never be able to hold onto the progress with the new body you have achieved.

Here is an example of how to calculate the amount of bodyfat you have and the amount of muscle you have.

EXAMPLE CALCULATION: This is for a person who weighs 150 pounds with 25% bodyfat, typical for many women.

Step 1) 100% –   25%   =   75%
                        (Bodyfat Percentage)   (Lean Mass Percentage)

Step 2) 75 / 100 = .75

Step 3) .75 x 150 = 112.5
So this person has 112.5 lb of lean mass at the start of the process and 37.5 lb of bodyfat.

This person's start point is:
Bodyweight: 150 lb
Lean Body Mass: 112.5 lb
Amount of Fat: 37.5 lb

Now lets say this person takes their calipers measurements two weeks later. This woman weighs 148 lb, but her bodyfat is now at 23%.

Step 1) 100%- 23%= 77%
So her lean mass has gone up to two percentage points.

Step 2) 77 / 100 = .77

Step 3) .77 x 148 = about 114 lb

So this person's new numbers are:
Bodyweight: 148 lb
Lean Body Mass: 114 lb
Amount of bodyfat: 34 lb
That's nearly a 10% reduction in bodyfat while the scale weight has only shifted two pounds!

NOW, IT'S TIME FOR YOUR CALCULATIONS DAY 1:

Take your measurements and fill in this chart to determine where you are at the starting point of your program.

Step 1)   100%   -   _____   =   _____
                       (your percentage of bodyfat)   (your lean mass %)

Step 2)   _____   /100 =   _____
             (your lean mass %)   (your lean mass as a decimal)

Step 3) _____ x _____ = _____
      (your current weight)   (your lean mass as a decimal)   (your lean mass in pounds)

Your start point is:

Bodyweight: _____ lb

Lean Body Mass: _____ lb

Amount of bodyfat: _____ lb

MAKE NEW CALCULATIONS ONCE A WEEK:

Perform this seven days after your start point. Then continue to record this data every week. Choose a day or the week where you can get a calipers test to continue to monitor your progress at regular intervals. Note that it's important to have the same person perform the calipers test as that's more accurate (in terms of your progress) than using different people for this test.

Step 1) 100% - _____ = _____

(your percentage of bodyfat)   (your lean mass %)

Step 2) _____ /100 = _____

(your lean mass %)   (your lean mass as a decimal)

Step 3) _____ x _____ = _____

(your current weight)   (your lean mass as a decimal)   (your lean mass in pounds)

Your start point is:
Bodyweight: _____ lb
Lean Body Mass: _____ lb
Amount of bodyfat: _____ lb

YOUR WEEK 3 CALCULATIONS:

Step 1) 100% - _____ = _____
                (your percentage of bodyfat)   (your lean mass %)

Step 2) _____ /100 = _____
                (your lean mass %)   (your lean mass as a decimal)

Step 3) _____ x _____ = _____
        (your current weight)   (your lean mass as a decimal)   (your lean mass in pounds)

Your start point is:
Bodyweight: _____ lb
Lean Body Mass: _____ lb
Amount of bodyfat: _____ lb

YOUR WEEK 4 CALCULATIONS:

Step 1) 100% - _____ = _____
                (your percentage of bodyfat)   (your lean mass %)

Step 2) _____ /100 = _____
                (your lean mass %)   (your lean mass as a decimal)

Step 3) _____ x _____ = _____
        (your current weight)   (your lean mass as a decimal)   (your lean mass in pounds)

Your start point is:
Bodyweight: _____ lb
Lean Body Mass: _____ lb
Amount of bodyfat: _____ lb

YOUR WEEK 5 CALCULATIONS:

Step 1) 100% - _____ = _____
             (your percentage of bodyfat)   (your lean mass %)

Step 2) _____ /100 = _____
             (your lean mass %)   (your lean mass as a decimal)

Step 3) _____ x _____ = _____
        (your current weight)   (your lean mass as a decimal)   (your lean mass in pounds)

Your start point is:
Bodyweight: _____ lb
Lean Body Mass: _____ lb
Amount of bodyfat: _____ lb

YOUR WEEK 6 CALCULATIONS:

Step 1) 100% - _____ = _____
             (your percentage of bodyfat)   (your lean mass %)

Step 2) _____ /100 = _____
             (your lean mass %)   (your lean mass as a decimal)

Step 3) _____ x _____ = _____
        (your current weight)   (your lean mass as a decimal)   (your lean mass in pounds)

Your start point is:
Bodyweight: _____ lb
Lean Body Mass: _____ lb
Amount of bodyfat: _____ lb

YOUR WEEK 7 CALCULATIONS:

Step 1) 100% - _____ = _____
                  (your percentage of bodyfat)   (your lean mass %)

Step 2) _____ /100 = _____
              (your lean mass %)   (your lean mass as a decimal)

Step 3) _____ x _____ = _____
        (your current weight)   (your lean mass as a decimal)   (your lean mass in pounds)

Your start point is:
Bodyweight: _____ lb
Lean Body Mass: _____ lb
Amount of bodyfat: _____ lb

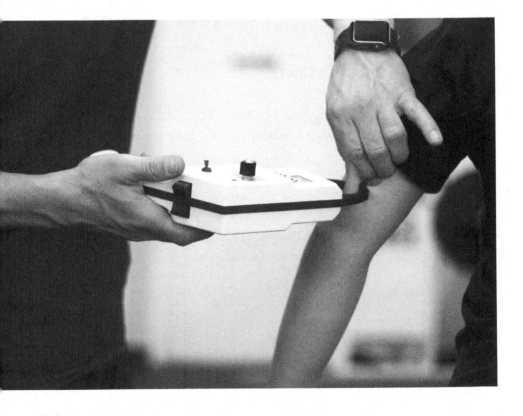

USE A SKIN-CALIPER TEST

These numbers are very important. You need to know that you are not losing muscle while you are losing fat. It's crucial when you do this that you have an accurate reading of your bodyfat or your numbers will be off. Many people use cheap bodyfat measurements that are inaccurate. I suggest a professional skin-caliper test because it's the easiest and least expensive way to get an accurate reading.

If you have the money and access, you can also get a hydrostatic bodyfat test, which provides an extremely accurate measure of bodyfat. But the latter isn't necessary unless you want to be hyper-vigilant. A skin-caliper test is nearly as accurate, far simpler and a great option to get you started.

SUPERHERO STORY:
Fat Loss Has No Pattern

⭐ In the video "22% of bodyfat in 6 weeks," one of the women, Claire, was losing a lot of bodyfat around her torso and for several days she felt as though she was looking funny and was really confused. So I explained to her that the areas that are lagging behind will pick up the pace quickly once the easy-to-lose areas are done losing all of their fat. Sure enough with another week the tough-to-lose places started to get smaller and then she relaxed into the process.

It's hard to wrap your brain around the idea that you don't lose fat evenly and it has a pattern all its own. Every person will not lose fat the same way, but in the end, if you follow this program, you will get the results you're seeking.

You should also take pictures of yourself, as I mentioned before. This is so you can also see your physical changes over time. It's important to understand that we do not choose where our bodies remove fat from first. Many times people will lose bodyfat and all of a sudden they see love handles they never saw before. They freak out and think this whole body-changing resolution is going terribly wrong and then they quit. This is why tracking your measurements is incredibly important. Retake your abdominal and other measurements each week and see how they've changed from the previous measurement. They may or may not be smaller, but at least you'll know.

Often, people lose bodyfat around their torso more quickly than the fat in their lower abdominal area. You may see a temporary period where this imbalance is noticeable to you more than anyone else. Keep working hard and stick to your plan. As certain areas of your body run out of fat to lose then your body will quickly attack your hard-to-lose areas. When you start attacking those hard-to-lose areas, you will start to see your body change almost daily. It's really empowering when you see yourself changing, because you realize that all your work is being realized.

SUPERHERO STORY:
Bodyfat Perspective

⭐ Below is a list of common bodyfat percentages of college student athletes from various sports.* It's important to understand that your goal is to lose bodyfat, not to get to a certain "idealized" goal. Note how much bodyfat percentages vary for many very successful athletes.

	MALE	FEMALE
Sprinting	8-10%	12-20%
Soccer	10-18%	13-18%
Swimmers	9-12%	14-24%
Tennis	12-16%	16-24%
Gymnastics	5-12%	10-16%
Distance running	5-11%	10-15%
Volleyball	11-14%	16-25%
Tennis	12-16%	16-25%
Shot Put	16-20%	20-28%
Ice/Field hockey	8-15%	12-18%
High/long jumpers	7-12%	10-18%
Baseball	12-15%	12-18%
Basketball	6-12%	20-27%
Football (backs)	9-12%	no data
Football (lineman)	15-19%	no data
Wrestling	5-16%	no data

* Moon J, Tobkin S, Smith A, Lockwood C, Walter A, Cramer J, Beck T, Stout J, "Anthropometric Estimates of Percent Bodyfat in NCAA Division I Female Athletes: A 4-Compartment Model Validation" J Str, Cond Res. 2009:23 (4) 1069-79

DON'T FEAR SUCCESS

I need to explain a phenomenon that over the 25-plus years I have trained I have seen play out time and time again. I call it "fear of success." This is a real phenomenon that is more difficult to deal with for many people than failure. If this is the first time you are seeing yourself achieve success in your body-transformation goal, then you are entering uncharted territory.

For instance, sometimes a compliment can backfire and send you longing for the place you were used to instead of being comfortable with your new body. If you believe you're starting to sabotage your progress, stop and regroup. Gather yourself and make a conscious effort to stop the sabotaging behavior. For example, you start to hit the candy jar you used to walk by, or you snack during the day. Or you begin to skip workouts and go out to eat instead.

Refocus and realize this journey is for you and no one else. Your fitness journey is the one of the few things in your life you can actually control. You can't control the economy, politics or what's going on in the world, but you can control what you put in your mouth and how much exercise you perform.

Below are a few suggestions I share with my clients to get them to stay on track throughout this transformation and beyond.

1) **Be positive.** Start every day before you get out of bed with a positive, one-line mantra such as: "I'm going to have a great day today!" Then smile. Don't underestimate this—it really helps start your day on a positive note.
2) **Realize you'll become an inspiration.** Remind yourself that your success will motivate others.
3) **Own your progress.** If you feel like you're going off track, then try saying something like, "Why not me?" Meaning why can't I be one of those people who is successful and reaches my goals? The beauty is that you are 100% in charge of you, and there will be nobody to thank or blame but you. Recall the enthusiasm you began this journey with and keep it going as you continue.

I believe that success breeds success. There are few things harder to do in life than to lose fat and keep it off. When you are in control of your body you should feel very confident and that shines from you in every interaction you have. People are always attracted to confidence, and it will open up unexpected doors at work and in your social life.

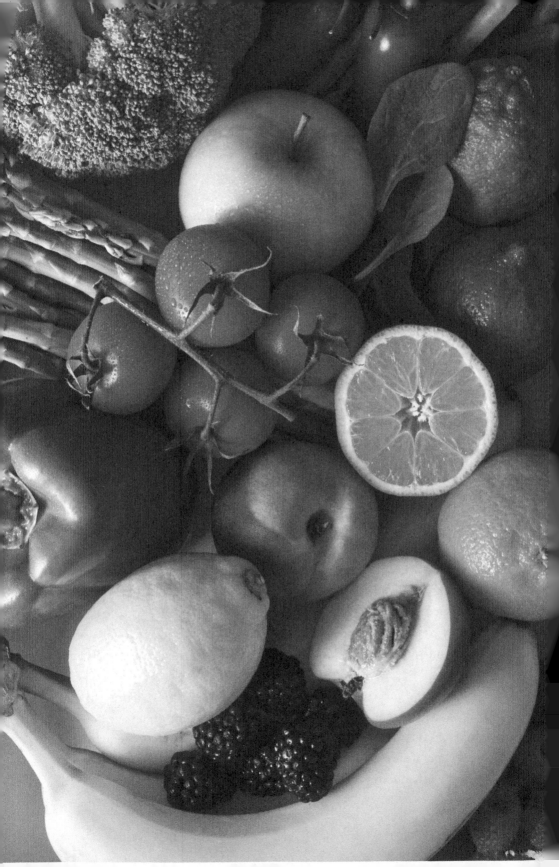

5

FOODS AND THEIR GLYCEMIC LOAD

Building a Smart Meal Plan by the Numbers

I've explained the importance of how macronutrients and foods impact your body's release of insulin. Now it's time for you to start to understand how to put together a nutrition program that will allow you to take advantage of all that I've learned over the years. The key is to choose foods that are of the proper numbers on the glycemic load (GL) index.

If a food has a score of more than 20 or so on the GL index, then you should cut the portion size down so it will fit in your zone for GL. That's true even if it's smaller than your hand measure would say. This is just a way of not limiting what you eat and getting bored on my nutrition program. If you do eat high GL foods, then just be careful to eat small or moderate portions.

MEAL SELECTION: KNOW YOUR SCORE

Your portion sizes will be either 1:2, 1:1.5 or 1:1, depending on your choices and goals. As a reminder, that means your protein choice should be of the hand-size that's right for you, and your carb choice should be based on the GL in a 1:2 ratio with the size of your protein, or 1:1.5 or 1:1 based on your goal.

Here's what's important: **The lower your overall GL score, the more you can eat.** It's a simple concept once you get used to checking GL scores.

For example, if you choose a skinless chicken breast, you could have twice the amount of a carbohydrate food that scores between 1-10 on the GL score (a 1:2 ratio). If you choose a carbohydrate that's between 11-20, then the carbohydrate and protein should be in a 1:1.5 ratio. Follow me on this part; if you didn't then re-read this section.

If you want to eat something that scores over 21, then cut the portion so it's the same size as your protein (a 1:1 ratio). For instance, if you choose a piece of salmon the size of your palm and first row of knuckles and you want a baked potato, which equals 36.4, then you need to cut the potato down to of your salmon. That ends up not being a lot of food when you are ...ng carbohydrates that are on the 21-and-over list. The concept is to try ...pick foods in the 1-10 list, so you can consume a larger volume of food. ...you choose to eat a secondary protein I would highly recommend that you ...ly choose carbs from the 1-10 part of the list so you can consume a reasonable volume of food. Volume is one of the keys to success on this program.

The good news: You will have a choice between many different daily meal plans and foods. Feel free to change it around, eat other foods you like, and make the nutrition program your own. **The most important thing to do is to try to stay within the 1:2 or 1:1.5 or 1:1 ratio that's right for you, and enjoy what you are eating.** Remember, salads are a free food as long as you use salsa (without oil) or lemon juice as a dressing. And don't add croûtons because they are a source of unwanted carbs.

GET A HANDLE ON YOUR PORTIONS AND RATIOS

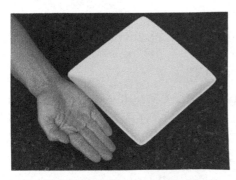

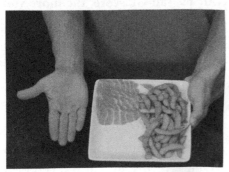

In this top photo you see a typically sized plate in comparison to a hand. Of course, you need to keep in mind that the hand-sized portion of a primary protein— or other size of protein—should be based on your hand. That's critical for determining portion size on my Superhero Nutrition program.

Here's a shot of my hand with an amount of salmon sashimi that's equal to my palm and first row of knuckles. Notice that the edamame is twice the size of the salmon because edamame is a carb that falls in the 1:2 ratio. This meal is perfect for fat-loss, but it may not be enough food if you're seeking to increase muscle mass. You can increase these amounts, proportionally, if your goal is to add bodyweight.

1:2 Ratio

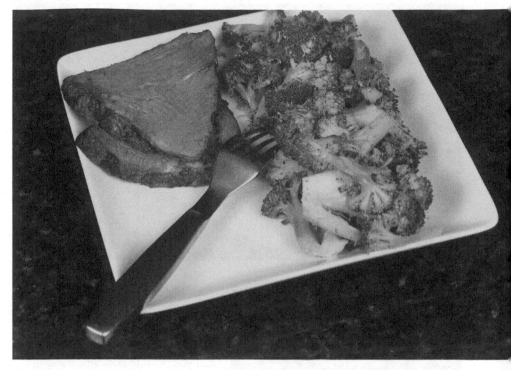

Here's what a full hand-sized portion of a primary protein looks like in comparison to double the amount broccoli, a low-glycemic-load carb choice for the 1:2 ratio for supporting muscle building without weight gain.

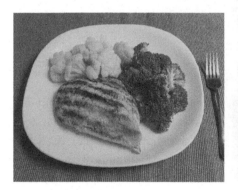 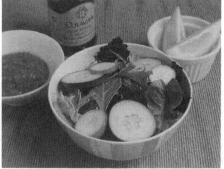

(Left to right) Split your low-glycemic-load carbs when you want to create more variety in your meals. You can always add a salad as a free food to any meal so long as you eat it with dressings that have virtually no impact on insulin: lemon, salsa or vinaigrette.

1:1.5 Ratio

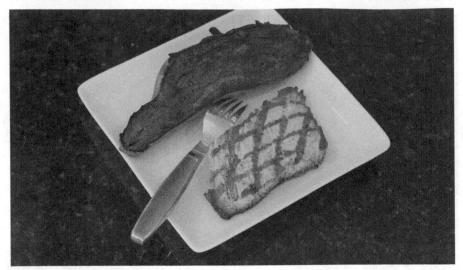

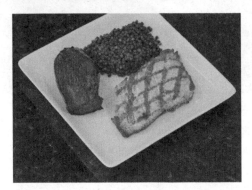

When you go with skinless chicken —a primary protein—and you want to add in other carbs, you can go with sweet potatoes and/or lentils. But you need to consume these in a 1:1.5 ratio because these foods trigger greater insulin release based on their glycemic load.

1:1 Ratio

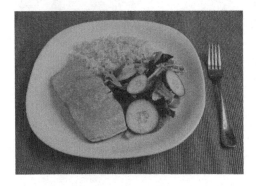

Sometimes you crave a carb that has a higher glycemic load. White rice is one of the foods on the 1:1 ratio list. Keep the portion of rice equal to your primary protein, but remember that you can consume as much salad as you want to make the quantity of food you consume satisfying.

When your goal is to burn fat while building or maintaining muscle mass, you can also add in healthy calories such as strawberries covered in 90% or higher dark chocolate that contains few grams of sugar.

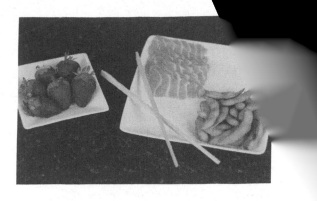

FOODS AND THEIR GL

This section provides the scientific specifics about the GL of individual foods, as consumed in typical (individual) quantities. That's much more important, as I've mentioned before, than how they measure on the unhelpful glycemic index. Before I get into the chart, though, I want to remind you of the parameters you should be searching for as you put together your daily meal plans.

But don't overthink this! I'm also going to provide you with several recipes and a 30-day meal plan to make this easy for you to follow and figure out for yourself. This section is merely to help you make choices beyond those I provide.

Some bullet points to keep you focused:

PRIMARY CARBOHYDRATE SELECTION

Any food that scores 10 or under is considered a primary carbohydrate. You can consume more of these than other carbs with higher GL scores.

SECONDARY CARBOHYDRATE SELECTIONS

Any foods that score between 11-20 on the list below. You need to consume about ¼ the quantity per serving or hand-size as a primary carb to control insulin release.

THE NEVER-EAT FOODS (UNLESS IT'S A CHEAT MEAL)

Avoid all foods above 20 on the list below unless you're consuming it during your two-hour, once-a-week cheat window, or you are following my rules for portion management.

an extensive list of the GLs of a variety of foods, separated by category. od you want to eat is not on this list, then just Google it. But make sure are giving you the GL and not the glycemic *index* for that food.

BEANS AND LEGUMES

These foods should be consumed liberally as your carb choice on my meal plan. The servings provide a large volume of food with little impact on insulin release. It's not a coincidence that many of these are also high in fiber, which not only supports health but also encourages fat loss.

BEANS AND LEGUMES	SERVING SIZE	GL
Soy beans	172 g (1 cup)	1.4
Peanuts	146 g (1 cup)	1.6
Green lentils	150 g (1 cup)	5
Mung beans	150 g (1 cup)	5
Red lentils	150 g (1 cup)	5
Butter beans	150 g (1 cup)	6
Yellow split peas	150 g (1 cup)	6
Lentils	198 g (1 cup)	7
Kidney beans	256 g (1 cup)	7
Black beans	150 g (1 cup)	7
Marrow fat beans, boiled and dried	150 g (1 cup)	7
Lima beans	241 g (1 cup)	7.4
Beans, dried and boiled	150 g (1 cup)	9
Pinto beans	171 g (1 cup)	11.7
Haricot and navy beans	150 g (1 cup)	12
Black eyed beans and peas	150 g (1 cup)	13
Chickpeas, boiled	240 g (1 cup)	13.3
Baked beans	253 g (1 cup)	18.2

VEGETABLES

Those that score a zero on the GL are essentially free foods that you can consume these the same way you take in salads when you want more food volume. These are your "free" foods when you want to eat more while losing fat. Keep in mind, though, that you shouldn't consume them between meals, either. Take in as much of these very low-calorie, low-GL foods with meals as you want. Those that score above zero should be consumed as your carbs choice, but you can make some adjustments in portion size based on the score. Remember, the lower the score, the more of that food you can consume, relative to the recommended serving size.

VEGETABLES	SERVING SIZE	GL
Broccoli, cooked	78 g (1/2 cup)	0
Cabbage, cooked	75 g (1/2 cup)	0
Spinach	30 g (1 cup)	0
Mushrooms	70 g (1 cup)	0
Cauliflower	100 g (1 cup)	0
Celery, raw	62 g (1 stalk)	0
Carrot, raw	15 g (1 large)	1
Tomato	123g (1 med)	1.5
Green peas	80 g	3
Pumpkin	80 g	3
Peas, frozen	72 g (1/2 cup)	3.4
Beets, canned	246g (1/2 cup)	9.6
Parsnip	78 g (1/2 cup)	11.6
Yam	150 g	13
Sweet corn on the cob	1 (small ear 6.5 inches)	14.0
Mashed potato	150 g	15
Yam	136 g (1 cup)	16.8
Sweet potato	150 g	17
Baked potato	150 g	18
French fries	150 g	22
Potato	213 g (1 med)	36.4

FRUITS

All fruits have an impact on insulin release because they contain sugar. That's true even though they often have plenty of fiber to mitigate that. You can include many of these fruits in your daily plans, but realize that you should stick to the recommended quantity that will keep the GL under 10 per serving. For those with scores above 10, you should reduce the serving size.

FRUITS	SERVING SIZE	GL
Plum	66 g (1 fruit)	1.7
Peach	98 g (1 med)	1.4
Grapefruit	123 g (1/2 fruit)	1.6
Cherries	120 g	5
Peaches, canned in juice	120 g	5
Strawberries	152 g (1 cup)	5
Sweet cherries, raw	117 g (1 cup)	6
Watermelon	120 g (1 fruit)	6
Apricot, raw	120 g	7
Peach	120 g (1 fruit)	7
Pear, canned in natural juice	120 g	7
Kiwi, w/ skin	76 g (1 fruit)	7
Apples, w/ skin	138 g (1med)	7.4
Grapes	92 g (1 cup)	9
Blueberries	150 g (1 cup)	9.6
Papaya	140 g (1 cup)	11.7
Pears	166 g (1 med)	12
Pineapple	120 g (1 fruit)	13
Watermelon	152 g (1 cup)	13.3
Orange	140 g (1 fruit)	18.2
Cantaloupe	177 g (1 cup)	7.8
Grapes	120 g	8
Peaches, canned in heavy/ light syrup	120 g	9
Apple, dried	60 g	10
Prunes	60 g	10

FRUITS	SERVING SIZE	GL
Papaya	120 g (1 fruit)	10
Pineapple, raw	155 g (1 cup)	11.9
Banana	118 g (1 med)	12.2
Pears, canned in pear juice	248 g (1 cup)	12.3
Mango	165 g (1 cup)	12.8
Figs, dried	60g	16
Pears, canned, light syrup	251 g (1 cup)	17.7
Raisins	43 g (small box)	20.5
Apricot, dried	130 g (1 cup)	23
Apricot, canned in light syrup (syrup is the issue)	253 g (1 cup)	24.3
Peaches, canned, heavy syrup (syrup is the issue)	262 g (1 cup)	28.4
Prunes	132 g (1 cup)	34.2
Dates	60g	42

NUTS

These foods are high in calories. But if you eat them in small quantities you can readily consume them with meals on my program. Consider adding them to salads or cooking with them. Note that they are NOT free foods that you can keep adding to salads (which are free foods). That's because nuts are high in calories despite their low GL.

NUTS	SERVING SIZE	GL
Walnuts	1oz	0
Almonds	1oz	0
Peanuts	1oz	1
Hazelnuts	1oz	1
Macadamia	1oz	1
Pecans	1oz	1
Cashews	1oz	2

DAIRY

Likely you know that many forms of dairy contain carbs, and virtually every form of dairy has some impact on insulin release. Nevertheless, some choices are still acceptable on my nutrition program. Note, interestingly, that skim and whole milk have the same GL, despite their difference in calories for the same quantity. That's due to the fact that the fat in whole milk slows insulin release. Again, calories aren't the only issue—it's also about insulin release and GL.

DAIRY	SERVING SIZE	GL
Yogurt, sweetened low fat	200 g	3
Milk, whole	244 g (1 cup)	4
Milk, skim	250 g (1 cup)	4
Mousse	50 g	4
Ice cream	72 g (1/2 cup)	6
Instant vanilla pudding	100 g	6
Custard (home made)	100 g	7
Instant chocolate pudding	100 g	7
Yogurt, reduced fat	200 g	7
Yogurt, plain	245 g (1 cup)	6.1
Soy milk	250 g	8
Pudding	100 g (1/2 cup)	8.4
Ice cream (lower fat)	76 g (1/2 cup)	9.4
Soy yogurt	200 g	13
Milk, condensed and sweetened	250 g	83

MEAT/PROTEIN

These foods contain calories and dietary fats, but they have no GL. Still, you need to consume them in the serving sizes that are right for you. Even though GL is crucial, calories begin to count after you've consumed a certain amount. Again, it's not a free-for-all. That's what my hand-size ratio is about: helping you balance serving size with GL.

MEAT/PROTEIN	SERVING SIZE	GL
Beef	3 oz	0
Chicken	3 oz	0
Eggs	1 large egg	0
Fish	3 oz	0
Lamb	3 oz	0
Pork	3 oz	0
Veal	3 oz	0
Deer venison	3 oz	0
Elk	3 oz	0
Buffalo	3 oz	0
Rabbit	3 oz	0
Duck	3 oz	0
Ostrich	3 oz	0
Shellfish	3 oz	0
Lobster	3 oz	0
Turkey	3 oz	0
Ham	3 oz	0

MIXED MEALS/CONVENIENCE FOODS

Every now and then you have little choice but to consume a meal on the go. When it's your only option, you don't need to feel as though you've fallen off your diet so long as you make good choices. Choose foods that have a low GL, and reduce portions to further reduce calories and the GL.

MIXED MEALS/CONVENIENCE FOODS	SERVING SIZE	GL
Chicken nuggets, frozen	100 g	7
Fish fingers	100 g	7
Pizza Super Supreme, thin and crispy (Pizza Hut)	100 g	9
Pizza Super Supreme (Pizza Hut)	100 g	9
Pies, party size beef	100 g	12
Pizza Vegetarian Supreme, thin and crispy (Pizza Hut)	100 g	12
Pizza, cheese	100 g	16
Sushi	100 g	19
Pizza, plain baked dough with Parmesan cheese and tomato sauce	100 g	22
Lean Cuisine, French chicken with rice	400 g	24
Spaghetti bolognaise	360 g	25
White bread with skim milk cheese	100 g	26
White and whole-meal wheat bread with peanut butter	100 g	26
White bread with butter	100 g	29
Kugel	150 g	31
Sirloin chop with mixed vegetables and mashed potato (home made)	360 g	35

NUTRITIONAL SUPPORT PRODUCTS

Many of these foods provide energy, but that often comes at the exp
burning bodyfat. Keep in mind that these foods contain calories and shou
be consumed in your fasting windows between meals. Also realize that m
of these products are designed for elderly or sick people who don't get in enou
calories to support optimal health.

NUTRITIONAL SUPPORT PRODUCTS	SERVING SIZE	GL
Choice vanilla	237 g	6
Glucerna, vanilla	237 g	7
Ensure Bar, chocolate fudge brownie	38 g	8
Resource Diabetic, French vanilla	237 g	8
Ensure Pudding, old-fashioned vanilla	113 g	9
Sustagen Instant Pudding, Vanilla powder mix	250 g	13
Ensure, vanilla	250 g	16
Ensure Plus, vanilla	237 g	19
Enercal Plus, made from powder	237 g	19
Resource Diabetic, Swiss chocolate	237 g	19
Ensure	237 g	19

REPLACEMENT PRODUCTS

...protein shakes are often designed to help bodybuilders and other athletes ...n weight. That often means both muscle mass and bodyfat. Keep in mind ...t you shouldn't take in calories in that 2-3–hour window before you exercise ...hen your goal is to reduce bodyfat. You can use protein shakes after workouts ...as part of your next meal, but you can also just as easily consume whole food meals that are rich in protein and provide more satiety.

MEAL REPLACEMENT PRODUCTS	SERVING SIZE	GL
Ultra Pure Protein shakes, cappuccino	250 g	1
Ultra Pure Protein shakes, Frosty chocolate	250 g	1
Ultra Pure Protein shakes, Strawberry shortcake	250 g	1
Ultra Pure Protein Shakes, Vanilla ice cream	250 g	1
Burn It Bars, chocolate deluxe	50 g	1
Burn It Bars, chocolate deluxe	50 g	2
Pure Protein bars, peanut butter	80 g	2
Designer Chocolate, sugar- free	35 g	3
Pure Protein Cookies, Choc-Chip Cookie Dough	55 g	3
Pure Protein Cookies, Peanut butter	55 g	3
Pure Protein bars, Chewy Choc-Chip	80 g	4
Pure Protein Cookies, coconut	55 g	4
Pure Protein bars, chocolate deluxe	80 g	5
L.E.A.N Products	40 g	6
Pure Protein bars, Strawberry Shortcake	80 g	6
Pure Protein bars, White chocolate mousse	80 g	6
Hazelnut and apricot bar	50 g	9

PASTAS/NOODLES

This category of foods is high in carbs and often high in fiber—the fiber often reduces the GL (as do pastas that contain meat or cheese due to fat content). Nevertheless, most of the foods in this category should be consumed infrequently or in small quantities when you're really craving them. They're a good option, though, for your once-a-week cheat meal.

PASTA/NOODLES	SERVING SIZE	GL
Tortellini, cheese	180 g	10
Ravioli, meat filled	180 g	15
Spaghetti, white	180 g	15
Spaghetti, whole meal	180 g	16
Fettuccine, egg	180 g	18
Instant noodles	180 g	19
Spaghetti, gluten-free	180 g	19
Capellini	180 g	20
Gluten free pasta	180 g	22
Linguine	180 g	22
Rice noodles	180 g	23
Macaroni	180 g	23
Udon noodles, plain	180 g	30
Corn pasta, gluten-free	180 g	32
Macaroni and cheese (Kraft)	180 g	32
Gnocchi	180 g	33
Rice pasta, brown	180 g	35

RICE/GRAINS

While many of these foods are considered to be low in calories, they're also high in fast-digesting carbs, which cause insulin release. And that bumps up their GL for fairly moderate portions. Add these foods in sparingly or save them for your weekly cheat meal.

RICE/GRAINS	SERVING SIZE	GL
Cracked wheat	150 g	12
Wheat, whole kernels	50 g (dry)	14
Rice, brown	150 g	18
Basmati	150 g	22
Rice, white (boiled)	150 g	23
Couscous	150 g	23
Long grain	150 g	23
Parboiled rice	150 g	26
Instant/puffed rice	150 g	29
Risotto rice	150 g	36
Jasmine rice	150 g	46

SOUPS

Many of these foods likely have a higher GL than you'd expect. Many soups also digest fairly quickly, providing satiety for a shorter period of time. While you can consume some soups that are very low (or zero) on the GL scale, you should be very aware of their GL before consuming them.

SOUPS	SERVING SIZE	GL
Noodle soup (traditional Turkish Soup with stock and noodles)	250 g	0
Tomato Soup	250 g	6
Minestrone, traditional, Country Ladle (Campbell's)	250 g	7
Lentil, canned	250 g	9
Split pea	250 g	16
Black bean	250 g	17
Green pea, canned (Campbell's)	250 g	27

BREADS

You CAN consume small servings of bread on my program, but note that they do have a GL and these serving sizes are fairly small (essentially one slice). When in doubt, cut out the breads. You can always enjoy them during your cheat meal. If you're going to eat bread during the process and you're unsure of the GL, then search for versions that are higher in fiber, but still keep portions moderate to small.

BREADS	SERVING SIZE	GL
Ezekiel bread	30 g	2
Rye bread	30 g	6
Sourdough rye	30 g	6
Sourdough wheat	30 g	8
Barley kernel bread	30 g	9
Barley flour bread	30 g	9
Oat bran bread	30 g	9
Buckwheat bread	30 g	10
Pita bread	30 g	10
Gluten free multigrain bread	30 g	10
White flour bread	30 g	10
Wonder, enriched bread	30 g	10
Cracked wheat bread	30 g	11
English muffin bread	30 g	11
Oat bread	30 g	12
Baguette, white	30 g	15
Bagel, white	70 g	25

SNACK FOODS/CONFECTIONARY

Yeah, you guessed it. You should avoid these foods while you're on the Superhero Nutrition program. I recommend that you eliminate most of these from your nutrition program altogether. Of course, you can include them as a cheat food if they're exactly what you're craving, but chips and popcorn, etc., are just not a good choice for calories or nutrition.

SNACK FOODS/ CONFECTIONERY	SERVING SIZE	GL
Fruity Bitz	15 g	4
Popcorn, plain	20 g	8
Potato crisps	50 g	11
Pretzels	30 g	16
Corn chips	50 g	17
Fruit Roll Up	30 g (1 snack)	24
Burger rings, BBQ	50 g	28

CANDY/SWEETS

You can eat these in very small quantities with your meals if this is what will keep you on my program. Still, most of these are best left for your two-hour cheat window once a week as they are low in beneficial nutrients, and high in unwanted sugar, often highly processed.

CANDY/SWEETS	SERVING SIZE	GL
Honey	1 Tbsp	3
Nutella	20 g	4
Dove Dark chocolate bar	37 g (1oz)	4.4
Peanut M&Ms	30 g (1oz)	5.6
Table sugar	2Tsp	7
Strawberry jam	2Tbsp	10.1
Twix bar	60 g	17
Life Savers, peppermint	30 g	21
Jelly beans	1 oz	22
Snickers bar	60 g (1/2 bar)	23

BAKED GOODS & CEREALS

These foods can count toward any of your three meals in the portions ⌐
below. Just make sure you don't overeat them. Those that rise above 10 sho⌐
consumed in smaller portions than the serving sizes on this list. And, of co.
beware of those that have a GL above 20.

BAKED GOODS & CEREALS	SERVING SIZE	GL
Popcorn	8 g (1 Cup)	2.8
Pumpernickel bread	26 g (1 Slice)	4.5
Taco shell	13 g (1 med)	4.8
Melba toast	12 g (4 rounds)	5.6
Oatmeal cookie	18 g (1 Large)	6
Oatmeal	117 g (1/2 Cup)	6.4
Plain scone	25 g (1 scone)	7
Corn tortilla	24 g (1 tortilla)	7.7
Wheat bread	28 g (1 slice)	7.7
Cornmeal-based taco shell	20 g	8
Graham crackers	14 g (2 sqrs)	8.1
Pound cake, Sara Lee	30 g (1 piece)	8.1
White bread	25 g (1 slice)	8.4
Rye bread, 100% whole	32 g (1 slice)	8.5
Apple muffin without sugar	60 g (1 muffin)	9
Cornmeal	13 g (1 cup)	9
Waffles	35 g (1 waffle)	10
Angel-food cake	28 g (1 slice)	10.7
Rye crisp crackers	25 (1 wafer)	11.1
Whole-wheat Mini Wheats	30 g (1 cup)	12
Raisin bran	30 g (1 cup)	12
Chocolate cake w/ chocolate frosting	64 g (1 slice)	12.5
Crumpet	50 g (1 piece)	13
Apple muffin with sugar	60 g (1 muffin)	13
Bran flakes	29 g (3/4 cup)	13.3
Cheerios	30 g (1 cup)	13.3
Oatmeal, instant	234 g (1 cup)	13.7

GOODS & CEREALS	SERVING SIZE	GL
...al K	30 g (1 cup)	14
...illa wafers	25 g	14
...ellogg's Special K	31 g (1 cup)	14.5
Bran muffin	57 g (1 muffin)	15
Pastry	57 g (1 pastry)	15
Pound cake	53 g (1 slice)	15
Banana cake/ no sugar	80 g (1 slice)	16
Buckwheat	150 g	16
Vanilla cake and vanilla frosting	64 g (1 slice)	16
Whole wheat pita	64 g (1 pita)	17
Blueberry muffin	57 g (1 muffin)	17
Plain sponge cake	63 g (1 slice)	17
Croissant	57 g (1 med)	17
Cake doughnut	47 g (1 doughnut)	17
Croissant butter	57 g (1 med)	17.5
Banana cake w/sugar	80 g (1slice)	18
Fruit Loops	30 g (1 cup)	18
Golden Grahams	30 g (1 cup)	18
Pikelets	40 g (1 piece)	18
Fiber Plus Bar	30 g (1 bar)	18
Waffle (home made)	75 g (1 waffle)	18.7
Angel food cake	50 g (1 piece)	19
Strawberry-iced cupcake	38 g (1 cupcake)	19
Chocolate cake (Betty Crocker)	111 g (1 slice)	20
Sweet corn	150 g	20
Coco Pops	30 g (1 cup)	20
Corn Chex	30 g (1 cup)	20.8
Cornflakes	28 g (1 cup)	21.1
Kaiser roll	57 g (1 roll)	21.2
Buckwheat pancakes	77 g (1 pancake)	22
Corn Pops	31 g (1 cup)	22.4
Rice Krispies	33 g (1 cup)	23

| --- | --- | --- |
Muselix	55 g (2/3 cup)	23.8
Vanilla (Betty Crocker)	111 g (1 slice)	24
Corn flakes	30 g (1 cup)	24
Donut (large glazed)	75 g (1 donut)	24.3
Raisin bran	61 g (1 cup)	24.4
Double chocolate Pop Tarts	50 g (1 pop tart)	25
French bread	64 g (1 slice)	29.5
Blueberry muffin	113 g (1 med)	30
Bran muffin	113 g (1 med)	30
Cornbread	60 g (1 piece)	30.8
Flan cake	70 g (1 slice)	31
Grape nuts	(1/2 Cup)	31.5
Bagel	89 g (1/4 in.)	33
Pancakes	80 g (1 pancake)	39

BEVERAGES

Few food groups are more easily consumed than beverages, as I mentioned earlier. Honestly, I recommend that you seek your calories from foods rather than beverages. These liquids tend to spike insulin without providing satiety, a terrible combination when you're trying to get lean and healthy.

BEVERAGES	SERVING SIZE	GL
Tomato juice	243 g (1 cup)	3.4
Soy milk	245 g (1 cup)	4
Yakult milk drink	65 g	6
Carrot juice (freshly made)	250 g	10
Grapefruit juice, unsweetened	250 g	11
Hot chocolate mix 28g	(1 packet)	11.7
Apple juice	248 g (1 cup)	11.9
Gatorade powder	16 g (.75 scoop)	12.5
Grapefruit juice, sweetened	250 g (1 cup)	13.4
Orange juice	249 g (1 cup)	14.25
Pineapple juice	250 g (1 cup)	14.7
Orange Fanta	250 g	23
Cranberry juice cocktail	153 g (1 cup)	24.5
Coca Cola	370 g (12 oz can)	25.2

SUGARS/SUGAR ALCOHOLS

Bodybuilders use sugar to drive insulin release to build muscle mass, but
you're a bodybuilder then insulin release is more likely to prevent bodyfat
being released from storage or, worse, cause more bodyfat to be stored. W
sugar alcohols have a low GL, you already know that I think they're bad for yc
I recommend avoiding sugar and sugar alcohols as much as possible. Save you.
sugar fix for your weekly cheat meal.

SUGARS/SUGAR ALCOHOLS	SERVING SIZE	GL
Lactitol	10 g	0
Litesse II, with polydextrose and sorbitol	10 g	0
Litesse III Ultra, with polydextrose and sorbitol	10 g	1
Xylitol	10 g	1
Blue Agave Cactus Nectar, high fructose	10 g	1
Fructose	10 g	2
Lactose	10 g	5
Glucose consumed with gum fiber	10 g	6
Maltitol, 25g Malbit CH (99% maltitol)	10 g	7
Sucrose	10 g	7
Glucose with 3g dried ginseng	10 g	8
Glucodex	10 g	8
Maltitol, 25g Maltidex 200 (50% maltitol)	10 g	9
Glucose	10 g	10
Honey	25 g	10

...ding the following groups of ethnic foods to show you how much they ... terms of GLs. As always, choose foods and portion sizes that fit the ...neters of your individualized program.

INDIGENOUS OR TRADITIONAL FOODS (AFRICAN)

AFRICAN	SERVING SIZE	GL
Gram dhal	50 g (dry)	1
Brown beans	50 g (dry)	6
Ga kenkey, from fermented cornmeal	150 g	7
Cassava, boiled with salt	100 g	12
Unripe plantain, raw	120 g	13
Gari	100 g	15
Yam	150 g	23
Maize meal porridge, unrefined	50 g (dry)	25
Maize meal porridge, refined	50 g (dry)	30
M'fino or morogo, wild greens	120 g	34
Maize meal porridge or gruel	50 g (dry)	41

INDIGENOUS OR TRADITIONAL FOODS (ARABIC OR TURKISH)

ARABIC OR TURKISH	SERVING SIZE	GL
Hummus	30 g	0
Turkish noodle soup	250 g	0
Stuffed grapevine leaves	100 g	5
Turkish bread, whole wheat	30 g	8
Kibbeh saynieh, lamb and burghul	120 g	9
Majadra	250 g	10
Turkish bread, white-wheat flour	30 g	15
Moroccan couscous	250 g	17
Lebanese bread (white, unleavened), hummus, falafel and tabbouleh	120 g	39

INDIGENOUS OR TRADITIONAL FOODS (ASIAN)

ASIAN	SERVING SIZE	GL
Lungkow bean thread	180 g	12
Glutinous rice ball with cut glutinous cake (mochi)	75 g	14
Rice gruel with dried algae	250 g	15
Rice noodles, fresh and boiled		
Lychee, canned in syrup (drained)	120 g	16
Mung Bean noodles, drained and boiled	180 g	18
Sushi	100 g	19
White rice and nonfat yogurt	150 g	19
Salted rice ball	75 g	20
Roasted rice ball	75 g	21
Rice vermicelli, Kongmoon	180 g	22
Soba noodles, instant, reheated	180 g	22
Rice noodles, dried and boiled	180 g	23
Rice cracker, plain	30 g	23
White rice with fermented soy bean	150 g	24
Udon Noodles	180 g	26
White rice with raw egg and soy sauce	150 g	26
White rice, dried sea algae and milk	300 g	26
Curry rice with cheese	150 g	27
White rice with pickled vinegar and cucumber	150 g	27
Glutinous rice flour with roasted soy bean	100 g	27
White rice with roasted ground soybean	150 g	29
White rice with instant miso soup	150 g	29
Glutinous rice cake with dried sea algae	75 g	32
White rice with low fat milk	300 g	32
Non-glutinous rice flour	100 g	34
Broken white rice	150 g	37
White rice with salted dried plum	150 g	39

ASIAN	SERVING SIZE	GL
White rice with sea algae rolled in sheet of toasted sea algae	150 g	39
Butter rice	150 g	40
White rice with dried fish strip (Okaka)	150 g	40
Curry rice	150 g	41
Low-protein white rice with dried sea algae	150 g	42
Glutinous rice	150 g	44
Jasmine white rice	150 g	46
Stir-fried vegetables, chicken and rice (home made)	360 g	55

INDIGENOUS OR TRADITIONAL FOODS (ASIAN INDIAN)

ASIAN INDIAN	SERVING SIZE	GL
Bengal gram dhal, chickpea	150 g	4
Black gram (Phaseolus mungo)	150 g	8
Barley (Hordeum Vulgare)	150 g	16
Amaranth, eaten with milk and nonnutritive sweetener	30 g	18
Bajra	75 g (dry)	29
Banana, nendra variety	120 g	31
Idli	250 g	36

INDIGENOUS OR TRADITIONAL FOODS (PACIFIC ISLANDER)

PACIFIC ISLANDER	SERVING SIZE	GL
Taro	150 g	4
Green banana/plantain	120 g	8
Yam	150 g	13
Sweet potato	150 g	17
Breadfruit	120 g	18

INDIGENOUS OR TRADITIONAL FOODS (CHAPPATI)

CHAPPATI	SERVING SIZE	GL
Dhokla	100 g	6
Green gram	150 g	6
Uppuma Kedgeree	150 g	6
Rajmah	150 g	6
Laddu	50 g	8
Cheela, Bengal gram, fermented batter	150 g	10
Cheela, green gram, fermented batter	150 g	10
Cheela, green gram	150 g	12
Tapioca, steamed	250 g	12
Cheela, Bengal gram	150 g	12
Chapatti, flour made from popped wheat, moth bean, and Bengal gram	60 g	14
Horse gram	150 g	15
Chapatti, wheat	60 g	21
Chapatti, flour from roller dried wheat, moth bean, and Bengal gram	60 g	23
Millet/Ragi, dehusked	150 g	23
Chapatti, flour from malted wheat, moth bean, and Bengal gram	60 g	25
Rice (Oryza Sativa)	150 g	26
Dosai	150 g	26
Poori	150 g	28
Upittu	150 g	28
Semolina, steamed	67 g (dry)	28
Green gram, whole with varagu	80 g (dry)	29
Lentil and cauliflower curry with rice	360 g	31
Chapatti, wheat flour, thin, with green gram dhal	200 g	32
Varagu	76 g (dry)	34
Pongal	250 g	35
Idli	250 g	36
Green Gram dhal with varagu	78 g (dry)	39

INDIGENOUS OR TRADITIONAL FOODS (AUSTRALIAN ABORIGINAL)

AUSTRALIAN ABORIGINAL	SERVING SIZE	GL
Acacia aneura, mulga seed, roasted, wet ground to paste	50 g	1
Castanospermum australe, blackbean seed sliced, soaked, pounded and baked	50 g	1
Araucaria bidwillii, bunya tree nut	50 g	7
Macrozamia communis, cycad palm seed	50 g	10
Acacia coriacea, desert oak, seed bread	75 g	11
Brush honey, sugar bag	30 g	11
Disoscorea bulbifera, cheeky yam, peeled, sliced, soaked, baked	150 g	12

INDIGENOUS OR TRADITIONAL FOODS (ISRAELI)

ISRAELI	SERVING SIZE	GL
Melawach and 15g locust bean	130 g	16
Melawach and 15g maize cob fiber	130 g	31
Melawach	115 g	35
Melawach and 15g lupin fiber	130 g	38

INDIGENOUS OR TRADITIONAL FOODS (PIMA INDIAN)

PIMA INDIAN	SERVING SIZE	GL
Acorns, stewed with venison	100 g	1
Mesquite cakes	60 g	1
Yellow teparies broth	250 g	8
Tortilla	60 g	9
White teparies broth	250 g	10
Lima beans broth	250 g	12
Corn hominy	150 g	12
Fruit leather	30 g	17
Cactus jam	30 g	18

INDIGENOUS OR TRADITIONAL FOODS (SOUTH AFRICAN)

SOUTH AFRICAN	SERVING SIZE	GL
Nopal	100 g	0
Pinto beans, boiled in salt water	150 g	4
Black beans	150 g	7
Wheat tortilla	50 g	8
Brown beans	150 g	9
Corn tortilla served with refried mashed pinto beans and tomato sauce	100 g	9
Corn tortilla, fried, with mashed potato, fresh tomato and lettuce	100 g	11
Arepa, made from dehulled high-amylose corn flour	100 g	11
Corn tortilla	50 g	12
Arepa, corn bread cake, made with corn flour	100 g	31
Arepa, made from ordinary dehulled dent corn flour	100 g	35

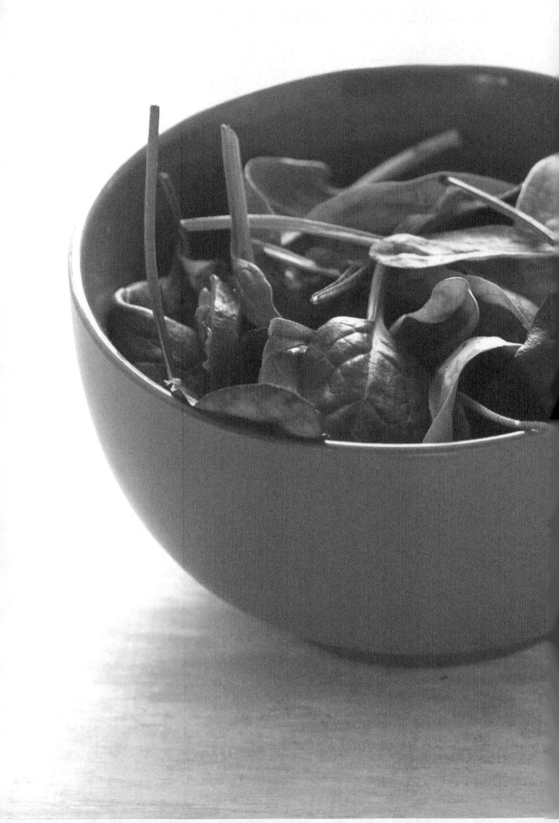

CHAPTER

6

YOUR 30-DAY MEAL PLAN

Satisfying Recipes That Will Keep You Lean

K nowing the GL for all these foods and the corresponding ratios for serving sizes will help you put your daily meal plans together. But I know you want more guidance. That's why I'm also providing a 30-day meal plan to give you a plan to help you construct a month-long nutrition program. These suggestions are based on basic foods and my recipes that come in the later chapters. I've divided the recipes into those for:

- Breakfast
- Lunch and dinner (which I consider interchangeable, regardless of whether you eat two or three meals a day)
- Desserts

One of the questions I get asked most often is, "What if I eat the same lunch or dinner five days or more in a row?"

My answer is that you can eat the same foods as often as you like, and it makes it easier to buy and prepare food. Of course, if you prepare food ahead of time you don't have to eat it the next day. You can store it in the refrigerator or freezer and create more variety while still reducing your prep time.

For instance, I love to get a serving of no-salt edamame and 8 oz of salmon sashimi multiple times a week. It's one of my favorite meals, and I don't get tired of it. And it also fits into my program. Here's how my plate looks (see page 88):

The salmon is the width and thickness of my palm and the first row of my knuckles. Then I double that amount in edamame (in the shell). If that leaves me hungry, then I either add more of these foods or include another food item that fits into my protein-to-carb ratio. Remember, a salad with salsa, lemon juice or oil-free vinaigrette is a free food, and you can also add that.

Sometimes I will add a serving of fruit with dark chocolate melted over it—you can find low-carb forms of dark chocolate if you like the taste (see page 91). It's very important that you eat enough at your meals that you don't feel hungry between meals and consider cheating. It's better to eat a little more during your meals than it is to "sneak" a bit in between. Remember, that's the primary tenet of my program: stopping the release of insulin release between meals is crucial to maximizing release of stored fat.

When you check out my recipes, you'll see examples such as "Steve's Famous Cauliflower Pizza." This may make you wonder about the protein content, but this main course is high in protein, which is in the cheese and cauliflower. Don't forget that many vegetables are high in protein, especially relative to their calories. That's yet another reason why they're low in GL.

Another question I frequently get asked is, "Should I eat kale—or some other 'healthy' food?" My answer is that you need to ask yourself if you like kale. My guess is that you don't if you're asking me that question. You should try different ways to prepare healthy foods to see if you can find a way that you enjoy them. If you still don't like them, then cut them out of your plan! Otherwise you'll start to resent what you're eating and that will likely sabotage your program.

When I started trying new foods with lower GLs, I found that I liked more and more foods from around the world. That's one of the reason why I've included so many foods from different cultures in the charts in Chapter 5. Many of these were unfamiliar to me until I began to search for ways to broaden my food choices while staying on my own program.

On the other hand, I know that some people couldn't care less about what they eat. They just eat what's in front of them, merely considering a meal to be a means to an end of biological necessity. I consider those people lucky, but I'm not one of them. I'm particular about what I eat. I look forward to each of my three meals a day, and I make sure that each one satisfies me because otherwise I'm going to have a long, miserable five hours between meals. But I want to stay on my own diet, and so I've found the foods and recipes that allow for that.

The next several pages includes an example of a three-meal-a-day program for 30 days. I've provided multiple examples of how you can put your 30-day program together with a lot of variety. Don't take this as a prescription that you need to follow food-by-food every day. Make the food choices that you like.

Superhero Nutrition for Everyone

⭐ My program will work for you even if you're on another restricted type of diet, you have health issues, or you need to avoid specific foods because of allergies. Here's a fairly lengthy list of other programs you can follow while integrating "Superhero Nutrition." That's one of the huge benefits of my program: It's compatible with many other food-restrictive programs. You can follow Superhero Nutrition at the same time that you follow any of these other plans:

Vegan
Vegetarian
Paleo
Low Carb
Atkins Diet
The Zone

Superhero Nutrition will also work if you want to cut out certain foods because of allergies, intolerances, or ethical or religious beliefs. These include:

Lactose intolerant
Kosher
Halal
Tree-nut allergy
Egg allergy
Milk allergy
Wheat allergy
Peanut allergy
Soy allergy
Corn allergy
Fruit allergy
Garlic allergy

Choose foods that fit your world. Then combine them with this program, and you'll lose more bodyfat than you thought possible. Just remember that timing is the most essential part of Superhero Nutrition and that the foods you choose are secondary. Of course, I don't recommend making poor nutritional choices. You will never get ripped eating sugar or large amounts of other carbohydrates, but you will still lose a substantial amount of bodyfat even if you are not strict with the 1:1.5 and 1:1 program I've laid out.

30-DAY SUPERHERO NUTRITION

Here's my day-by-day example of how to implement and follow my program. Again, you should make the adaptations that are right for you based on the foods you like, and/or those that are on your program. Your hand will do the calorie counting for you, so if you stick to that, you'll always hit the calorie count your body needs.

DAY 1

Drink 1 oz of apple-cider vinegar and 12 oz of water before EVERY meal

Breakfast:

- 1 Large egg with 2 egg whites with tomatoes
- 1 Large apple

Lunch:

- Green salad with cut tomatoes, with your choice of dressing
- Chicken/quinoa bowl *(recipe on page 171)*
- 1 Large grapefruit

Dinner:

- Green salad with your choice of dressing
- Grilled halibut
- Broccoli
- Cauliflower rice *(recipe on page 188)*

Superhero Nutrition—Portion Size

⭐ Some foods or recipes you'll make will come out larger than your hand. But still use your hand metric for your portions—and only eat that amount. After all, it's difficult to determine how many cooked eggs are as big as your hand. That's better determined after cooking than before. And the size of everyone's hand differs.

In my 30-day program, I provide guidance on the foods and portion sizes that may be right for you based on my hand size. But you should adapt these to your own needs and hand size.

DAY 2

Drink 1 oz of apple-cider vinegar and 12 oz of ***water*** *before EVERY*

Breakfast:

- Quinoa nut bowl *(recipe on page 162)*
- 2 hard boiled egg whites (not the yolk)

Lunch:

- Grapefruit sushi *(recipe on page 178)*
- 1 Banana with 90% or higher dark chocolate dripped on
  (use 1 to 2 cubes of chocolate)

Dinner:

- Green salad with your choice of dressing
- Beef stew *(recipe on page 182)*
- Cauliflower mashed potatoes *(recipe on page 186)*

DAY 3

Drink 1 oz of apple-cider vinegar and 12 oz of water before EVERY meal

Breakfast:

- Healthy avocado toast *(recipe on page 191)*

Lunch:

- Green salad with your choice of dressing
- All-American turkey burger on a green salad, can add Wellebee's
  Honey Ketchup *(recipe on page 184)*
- Sweet potato baked French fries *(recipe on page 193)*

Dinner:

- Grilled vegetable salad with 1 tablespoon of goat cheese you
  can spread on the vegetables
- Grilled butterfish
- Cauliflower mashed potato *(recipe on page 186)*
- Chocolate fondue *(recipe on page 197)*

z of apple-cider vinegar and 12 oz of water before EVERY meal

st:

ice Ezekiel bread with nut butter and half a sliced banana on *top*

Medium apple

Lunch:

- Green salad with your choice of dressing
- Chicken stir-fry (cauliflower rice instead of rice) *(recipe on page 172)*
- 1 cup of sliced watermelon

Dinner:

- Green salad with your choice of dressing
- Grilled chicken breast
- Steamed mix vegetables
- Zucchini spaghetti *(recipe on page 190)*

DAY 5

Drink 1 oz of apple-cider vinegar and 12 oz of water before EVERY meal

Breakfast:

- Banana beet bowl *(recipe on page 161)*

Lunch:

- Chinese chicken salad with Asian salad dressing *(recipe on page 173)*
- Cauliflower buffalo wings *(recipe on page 186)*

Dinner:

- Grilled salmon
- Cooked spinach
- Steamed zucchini
- 1 cup of berries

DAY 6

Drink 1 oz of apple-cider vinegar and 12 oz of water before EVERY meal

Breakfast:

- Yogurt 6 oz (your choice, keep the sugar under 7 grams)
- 2 oz Blueberries
- 3 Hard boiled eggs (I eat 1 whole egg and 2 egg whites)

Lunch:

- Green salad with your choice of dressing
- Spicy tuna cucumber roll; use low sodium soy sauce
  (in Japan they touch their sushi with the soy sauce; in the United States we bathe our sushi in it. Lets act more like the Japanese and go easy on the soy sauce. Be aware soy sauce has gluten but a gluten-free version is available).
- 1.5 cups Edamame, boiled no salt

Dinner

- Green salad with your choice of dressing
- Chicken and cauliflower casserole *(recipe on page 173)*
- Sweet potato baked French fries *(recipe on page 193)*

DAY 7

Drink 1 oz of apple-cider vinegar and 12 oz of water before EVERY meal

Breakfast:

- Protein pancakes *(recipe on page 154)*
- 1 medium apple

Lunch:

- Green salad with your choice of dressing
- Grapefruit sushi *(recipe on page 178)*

Dinner:

- Green salad with your choice of dressing
- Beef stew (scoop out 2 cups as a serving) *(recipe on page 183)*
- Cauliflower mashed potatoes (1 serving) *(recipe on page 186)*

DAY 8

Drink 1 oz of apple-cider vinegar and 12 oz of water before EVERY meal

Breakfast:

- Banana beet bowl *(recipe on page 161)*

Lunch:

- Salmon sashimi salad
- 1 Large orange

Dinner:

- Green salad with your choice of dressing
- Grilled filet mignon
- Sautéed vegetables
- Cauliflower mashed potatoes *(recipe on page 186)*
- 1 Block 90% or higher chocolate melted over 4 strawberries *(recipe on page 203)*

DAY 9

Drink 1 oz of apple-cider vinegar and 12 oz of water before EVERY meal

Breakfast:

- Quinoa nut bowl (eat 1 or 2 servings from the recipe I've included) *(recipe on page 162)*

Lunch:

- 1 Grilled artichoke
- Grilled chicken breast plate *(recipe on page 171)*

Dinner:

- 1 Large cut tomato with your choice of dressing
- Baked halibut
- Cauliflower French fries *(recipe on page 185)*
- Chocolate protein pudding *(recipe on page 198)*

DAY 10

Drink 1 oz of apple-cider vinegar and 12 oz of water before EVERY me

Breakfast:

3 Eggs (1 whole egg and 2 egg whites) with 2 oz salmon

Lunch:

- Green salad with your choice of dressing (something I like to do is make my salad and then put it on top of the pizza)
- Steve's Famous Cauliflower Pizza *(recipe on page 169)*
- Fruit of your choice

Dinner:

- Green salad with your choice of dressing
- Non-fried non-rice chicken bowl *(recipe on page 175)*
- Steamed broccoli
- Peanut butter banana ice cream *(recipe on page 199)*

DAY 11

Drink 1 oz of apple-cider vinegar and 12 oz of water before EVERY meal

Breakfast:

- Cottage cheese 6 oz

Add in

- 2 oz Blueberries
- ½ Banana (sliced)

Lunch:

- Grilled vegetable salad with 2 tablespoons of goat cheese (optional)
- Cauliflower steak *(recipe on page 188)*
- Salmon fillet

Dinner:

- Chinese stir-fry with shrimp *(recipe on page 193)*
- Cauliflower rice *(recipe on page 188)*
- Strawberry ice cream *(recipe on page 199)*

...oz of apple-cider vinegar and 12 oz of water before EVERY meal

...ast:

...een smoothie (I have it listed under desserts but all my desserts could ...e eaten anytime) *(recipe on page 200)*

Lunch:
- Lettuce-wrapped chicken *(recipe on page 174)*
- Acai bowl *(recipe on page 202)*

Dinner:
- Green salad with your choice of dressing
- Black cod
- Cauliflower buffalo wings *(recipe on page 186)*
- Steamed green beans

DAY 13

Drink 1 oz of apple-cider vinegar and 12 oz of water before EVERY meal

Breakfast:
- Cottage cheese 6 oz 0% fat

Mix in
- 2 oz Pomegranate seeds
- 2 oz Grapes

Lunch:
- Green salad with your choice of dressing
- Spaghetti squash pasta *(recipe on page 189)*
- Grilled brocollini

Dinner:
- Green salad with 1 cut tomato and your choice of dressing
- Black cod
- Grilled bell peppers
- Asparagus
- Peanut butter banana ice cream *(recipe on page 199)*

DAY 14

Drink 1 oz of apple-cider vinegar and 12 oz of water before EVERY meal

Breakfast:

- Chocolate shake *(recipe on page 159)*
- Poached egg (or prepare any way you like)

Lunch:

- Green salad with your choice of dressing
- Spicy tuna non-roll *(recipe on page 179)*
- Edamame
- Brussels sprouts

Dinner:

- Green salad with your choice of dressing
- Lean grilled steak
- Cauliflower buffalo wings *(recipe on page 186)*
- Sweet potato baked French fries *(recipe on page 193)*
- Chocolate protein pudding *(recipe on page 198)*

DAY 15

Drink 1 oz of apple-cider vinegar and 12 oz of water before EVERY meal

Breakfast:

- 1 Large apple with 2 tablespoons organic peanut butter
- 1 0% fat 6 oz Greek yogurt with 1 oz pineapple and 1 oz raspberries

Lunch:

- Chinese food *(recipe on page 193)*
- Acai bowl *(recipe on page 202)*

Dinner:

- Green salad with your choice of dressing
- Spaghetti squash pasta *(recipe on page 189)*
- Black beans
- 1 Large artichoke
- Chocolate covered fruit *(recipe on page 203)*

DAY 16

Drink 1 oz of apple-cider vinegar and 12 oz of water before EVERY meal

Breakfast:

- Fruit salad 6 oz
- Protein pancakes *(recipe on page 154)*

Lunch:

- Steak vegetable salad with your choice of dressing (I prefer balsamic with this dish) *(recipe on page 181)*
- Cauliflower French fries *(recipe on page 185)*

Dinner:

- Vegetable salad with your choice of dressing
- Grilled piece of fish of your choice
- Eggplant
- Zucchini
- Strawberry ice cream *(recipe on page 199)*

DAY 17

Drink 1 oz of apple-cider vinegar and 12 oz of water before EVERY meal

Breakfast:

- Chocolate vegan granola bar (1 serving) *(recipe on page 160)*
- Piece of fruit of your choice

Lunch:

- Green salad your choice of dressing (I like to put the salad on the pizza)
- Steve's Famous Cauliflower Pizza *(recipe on page 169)*
- Quinoa nut bowl *(recipe on page 162)*

Dinner:

- Green salad with chickpeas and your choice of dressing
- Grilled breast of chicken
- Steamed kale
- Steamed carrots
- Greek yogurt smoothie *(recipe on page 200)*

DAY 18

Drink 1 oz of apple-cider vinegar and 12 oz of water before EVERY meal

Breakfast:

- Yogurt parfait (1 Serving) *(recipe on page 155)*
- 2 Eggs

Lunch:

- Grilled bell peppers
- Grilled salmon
- Hummus
- Cauliflower rice *(recipe on page 188)*

Dinner:

- Green salad with grape tomatoes and your choice of dressing
- Piece of lean beef
- Cauliflower mashed potatoes *(recipe on page 186)*
- Green beans

DAY 19

Drink 1 oz of apple-cider vinegar and 12 oz of water before EVERY meal

Breakfast:

- 1 Slice Ezekiel bread with guacamole
- 1 Large grapefruit

Lunch:

- 2 or 3 Lettuce-wrapped chicken *(recipe on page 174)*
- Cauliflower steak *(recipe on page 188)*
- Chocolate protein pudding *(recipe on page 198)*

Dinner:

- Green salad with your choice of dressing
- Fish dishes

DAY 20

Drink 1 oz of apple-cider vinegar and 12 oz of water before EVERY meal

Breakfast:

- 1 Egg, 2 egg whites with 2 oz mushrooms, 2 oz tomatoes, 2 oz eggplant mixed in

Lunch:

- Non-fried non-rice chicken bowl *(recipe on page 175)*
- Green smoothie *(recipe on page 200)*

Dinner:

- Green salad with your choice of dressing
- Broccoli chicken *(recipe on page 174)*
- Chocolate protein pudding *(recipe on page 188)*

DAY 21

Drink 1 oz of apple-cider vinegar and 12 oz of water before EVERY meal

Breakfast:

- Healthy pancakes *(recipe on page 157)*
- 1 Scrambled egg with 1 added egg white

Lunch:

- Grapefruit sushi *(recipe on page 178)*
- Chocolate vegan granola bar *(recipe on page 160)*

Dinner:

- Grilled vegetable salad
- Grilled fillet mignon
- Medium sweet potato
- Peanut butter banana ice cream *(recipe on page 199)*

DAY 22

Drink 1 oz of apple-cider vinegar and 12 oz of water before EVERY meal

Breakfast:

- 6 oz plain Greek yogurt 0% fat
- Add 2 oz frozen blueberries (this tastes like dessert)

Lunch:

- Salad with yellowtail and salmon sashimi in it, use the dressing of your choice or just low-sodium soy sauce.

Dinner:

- Green salad with your choice of dressing
- Chicken plate

DAY 23

Drink 1 oz of apple-cider vinegar and 12 oz of water before EVERY meal

Breakfast:

- Vegan protein shake *(recipe on page 159)*

Lunch:

- Green salad with your choice of dressing
- Grilled tuna
- Steamed spinach
- Brussels sprouts

Dinner:

- Green salad with your choice of dressing
- Spaghetti squash pasta with turkey meat sauce *(recipe on page 189)*

DAY 24

Drink 1 oz of apple-cider vinegar and 12 oz of water before EVERY meal

Breakfast:

- Banana with 2 tablespoons organic almond butter

Lunch:

- Chicken and cauliflower casserole *(recipe on page 173)*

Dinner:

- All-American turkey burger *(recipe on page 184)*
- Sweet potato baked French fries *(recipe on page 193)*
- Chocolate protein pudding *(recipe on page 188)*

DAY 25

Drink 1 oz of apple-cider vinegar and 12 oz of water before EVERY meal

Breakfast:

- Spinach and cheddar quiche *(recipe on page 157)*

Lunch:

- Yellowtail sashimi salad
- Edamame, no salt

Dinner:

- Green salad with your choice of dressing
- Beef stew *(recipe on page 182)*

DAY 26

Drink 1 oz of apple-cider vinegar and 12 oz of water before EVERY meal

Breakfast:

- 1 Slice Ezekiel bread with nut butter and ½ sliced banana on top

Lunch:

- Grilled chicken plate

Dinner:

- Green salad with your choice of dressing
- Grapefruit sushi *(recipe on page 178)*

DAY 27

Drink 1 oz of apple-cider vinegar and 12 oz of water before EVERY meal

Breakfast:

- Healthy pancakes *(recipe on page 157)*

Lunch:

- Chinese chicken salad *(recipe on page 171)*
- Edamame
- Zucchini

Dinner:

- Spaghetti squash with turkey meat sauce *(recipe on page 189)*
- Banana ice cream *(recipe on page 198)*

DAY 28

Drink 1 oz of apple-cider vinegar and 12 oz of water before EVERY meal

Breakfast:

- Chocolate shake *(recipe on page 159)*

Lunch:

- Broccoli chicken *(recipe on page 174)*

Dinner:

- Green salad with your choice of dressing
- Filet mignon
- Asparagus
- Sauteed mushrooms
- Sauteed spinach

DAY 29

Drink 1 oz of apple-cider vinegar and 12 oz of water before EVERY meal

Breakfast:

- Banana beet bowl *(recipe on page 161)*

Lunch:

- Broccoli chicken *(recipe on page 174)*
- 2 Portions of cauliflower rice *(recipe on page 188)*

Dinner:

- Green salad with your choice of dressing
- Grilled cod
- Sweet potato
- Brussels sprouts

DAY 30

Drink 1 oz of apple-cider vinegar and 12 oz of water before EVERY meal

Breakfast:

- Fruit salad
- Vegan protein shake *(recipe on page 159)*

Lunch:

- Steve's Famous Cauliflower Pizza with green salad on top *(recipe on page 169)*

Dinner:

- Green salad with your choice of dressing
- Grilled chicken breast
- Green beans
- Cauliflower
- Chocolate shake *(recipe on page 159)*

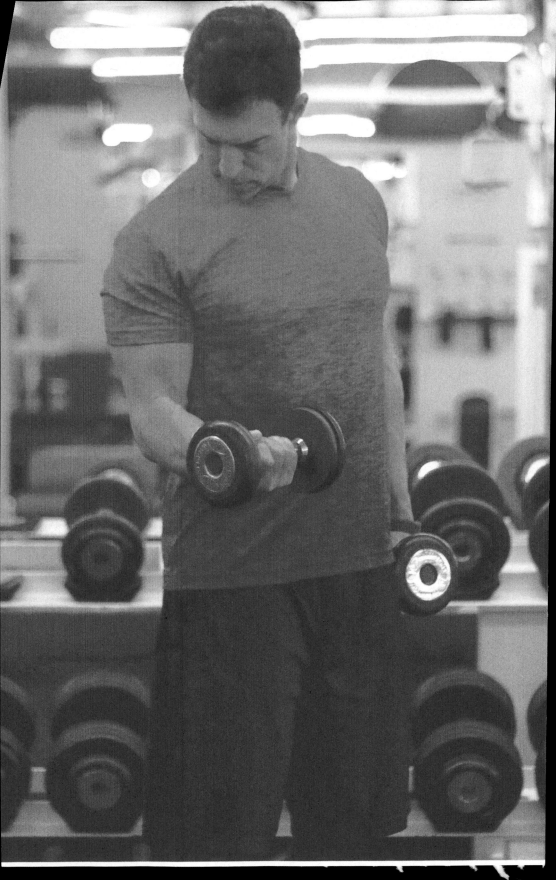

7

SUPERHERO WORKOUTS FOR FAT LOSS

Becoming a Fat-Burning Machine

One question you may have is: "What should my workouts be like?" While I've addressed that earlier to a certain extent, I'd like to give you more information on that ahead of publishing my next book, *Superhero Training*. In addition to what I'm providing below, I'd also like to refer you to my previous books, which will help you in the meantime.

What follows is an introductory three-day-a-week sample workout program to give you an idea of what I'm talking about. You can find much more detailed workouts in my training books. The movements in my books are very unique and are all photographed and explained in tremendous detail.

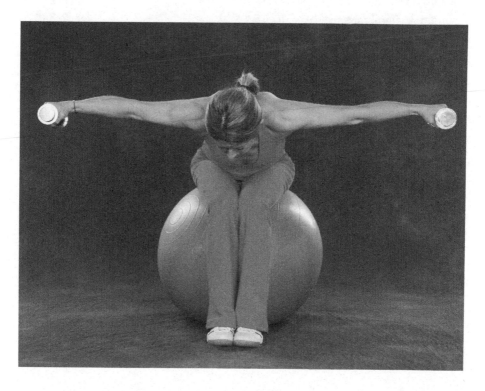

Monday

Warm up for five minutes on a treadmill, elliptical, bike or whatever cardio you'd like to do. Make sure you do not warm up by stretching when your muscles are cold. If you stretch them at this time, you could cause a major injury. Muscle tissue needs to be warmed up before it can be fully elongated safely.

On Monday, you'll target your legs with classic moves, and you'll hit four of your upper bodyparts (chest, back, shoulders, triceps) for one exercise each. Then you'll finish with abs and core training.

	REPETITIONS	WEIGHTS	SETS
Leg extensions	10-15	(whatever you can do comfortably for 80% and work the last 20%)	2-3
Leg curls	10-15	"	2-3
Squats	10-15	"	2-3
Calf raises	10-20	"	2-3
Dumbbell flat-bench flyes	10-15	"	2-3
Seated rows	10-15	"	2-3
Dumbbell lateral raises	10-15	"	2-3
Triceps pressdowns	10-15	"	2-3
Abdominals crunches	20	0	2-3
Bicycles	20	0	2-3
Planks	5	0	30 seconds per set

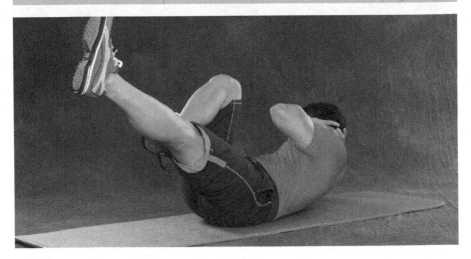

Wednesday

After a five-minute warm-up, you'll train your lower body using a variety of different moves than what you did on Monday—you can vary your leg curls by using an alternative version, such as one leg at a time. Then you'll work muscles in your upper body, targeting back, shoulders, chest and biceps. Again, abs and core should come at the end of your training session.

	REPETITIONS	WEIGHTS	SETS
Abduction machine	10-15	(whatever you can do comfortably for 80% and work the last 20%)	2-3
Adduction machine	10-15	"	2-3
Front lunges	10-15	"	2-3
Leg curls	10-15	"	2-3
Lat pulldowns	10-15	"	2-3
Dumbbell bent over rear deltoid flyes	10-15	"	2-3
Dumbbell incline flyes	10-15	"	2-3
Standing dumbbell curls	10-15	"	2-3
Abdominals			
Bicycles	10-20	0	2-3
Hip lifts (back flat, legs up above head, lift up 3-6 inches)	10-20	0	2-3
Side plank	5 per side	0	30 seconds each side per set

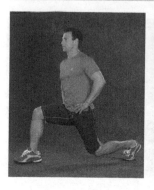
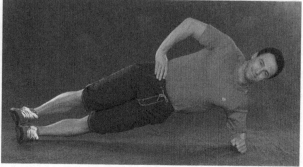

Friday

Again, you'll perform a five-minute cardio warm-up. Then you'll target your upper body before your lower on this third training session of the week, hitting all five upper-body muscle groups (back, chest, shoulders, triceps and biceps). Then you'll train your legs and give them two days of rest before your next weight workout on Monday. I incorporate abs exercises into all of my weight-training workouts on this three-day-a-week program.

	REPETITIONS	WEIGHTS	SETS
Push-ups	10-15	(what ever you can do comfortably for 80% and work the last 20%)	2-3
Dumbbell One-arm rows	10-15 per side	"	2-3
Dumbbell kickbacks	10-15	"	2-3
Dumbbell shoulder presses	10-15	"	2-3
Dumbbell hammer curls	10-15	"	2-3
Leg extensions	10-15	"	2-3
Leg curls	10-15	"	2-3
Leg presses	10-15	"	2-3
Abdominals:			
Standing side raises	10-15	"	2-3
Hip lifts	10-20	0	2-3
Crunches	10-20	0	2-3

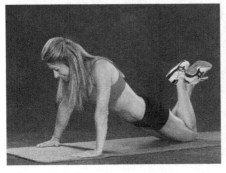
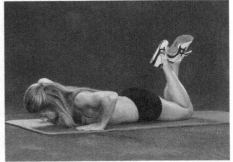

CARDIO AND WEIGHT TRAINING SCHEDULE

In addition to weight training three times a week, you should also perform a minimum of three cardio sessions each week. Preferably, you should do these on days when you aren't lifting weights. By offsetting cardio and lifting days you will be exercising six days a week. If you want to do more than three days a week of cardio, then you can overlap workout and cardio days. Take a look at my recommendations in Chapter 3.2 to remind yourself when to eat before and after cardio to maximize fat loss.

The purpose is that you'll be working out six days a week to keep revving your metabolism and burning bodyfat. Of course, the level of intensity for these training sessions depends on your current level of fitness. Don't go all-out with every set, rep and cardio session. Follow my guidelines for intensity regardless of your level of fitness. That's crucial because you're also adapting to a different pattern of eating, which is even more critical.

WEEKLY SPLITS

Here are a few different ways you can put together your training program. I realize that you have a busy life, and one of these options may work better for you than others. My goal is to get you to do six workouts a week, regardless of when you perform them. First, is my ideal training split, and then I provide a couple examples of how you can change this up to fit your needs. Feel free to come up with your own program if these don't fit your lifestyle.

Superhero Workout—My Ideal Program Split

Monday:	Weights
Tuesday:	Cardio
Wednesday:	Weights
Thursday:	Cardio
Friday:	Weights
Saturday:	Cardio
Sunday:	Rest

Superhero Workout—An Alternative

Monday: Weights followed by cardio

Tuesday: Rest

Wednesday: Weights

Thursday: Cardio

Friday: Weights followed by cardio

Saturday: Rest

Sunday: Rest

Superhero Workout—Another Alternative

Monday: Cardio in the morning; weights later in the day

Tuesday: Rest

Wednesday: Cardio (whatever time of day)

Thursday: Weights (my Wednesday workout)

Friday: Cardio (whatever time of day)

Saturday: Weights (my Friday workout)

Sunday: Rest

So here are my most crucial guiding principles for putting together a workout program that works for you:
1) Perform three weight-training sessions a week
2) Perform at least three cardio sessions a week
3) Try to create a rest day between each of your three weight workouts each week
4) But perform the weight workouts back-to-back rather than skipping one
5) Back off on any form of exercise for a day or two if you feel overly sore or over-trained

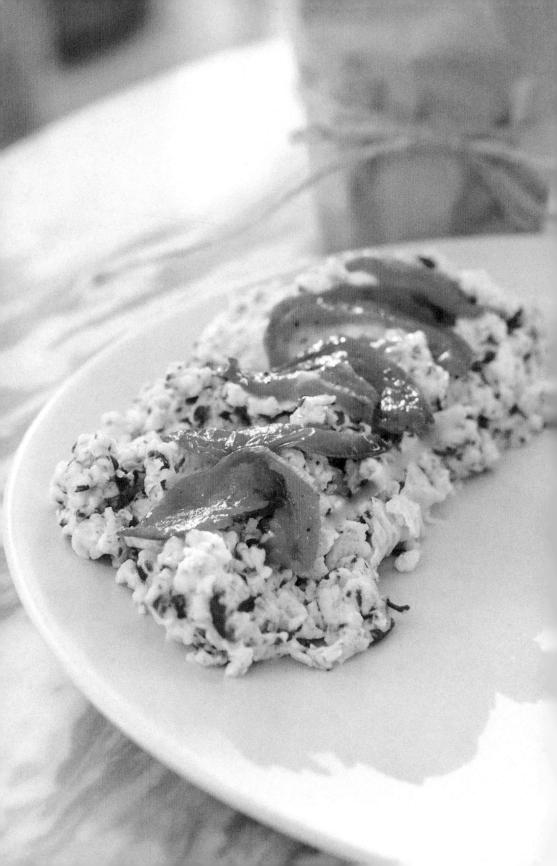

8

OWN THE DAY

Breakfast Recipes for a Great Start

How you start the morning sets the tone for the entire day. Don't waste the opportunity to make the most of it.

Breakfast is the first meal of the day, and its timing is critical. Your body would rather have you eat food after a workout than before. Many of us are accustomed to waking up and eating, which is okay if you don't plan to train. The only time you would eat breakfast before you train is if you have at least a two-hour window from breakfast until your workout.

Realize that once you're done eating, you will be left with two more meals for the day. When you wake up, have coffee or tea if you want, but don't add anything to it that has over 10 calories total. If you take in over 10 calories, you will spike your insulin levels.

Let's face it: Many of us don't have a lot of time in the morning before our workouts anyway. So if you're not hungry first thing in the morning, you can wait to eat about an hour or two after you wake up. You will be burning fat the entire time you're up, until you take your first bite of food. What is key is to then have at least a five-hour break before the next time you eat.

PICK YOUR MEAL TIMING FOR YOUR LIFESTYLE

Carefully planning your meal times is essential to making my nutrition plan work for you. It is also important to be honest with yourself about what meals you like most. Are you a breakfast, lunch or dinner person? You can choose to eat about the same amount of food at each sitting, but people who love breakfast might choose to eat more at breakfast and less at lunch and dinner. So keep your personal preferences in mind as you build each day's schedule.

Do not force yourself to become somebody you're not. Being true to when and what you like to eat is essential in making this nutrition plan a long-term lifestyle change. Due to lifestyle a lot of people do not have the time to eat a large sit-down breakfast. If that's the case for you, then there are still plenty of items included in this chapter that you can eat on the run.

I've also added breakfast options I like when you have time to actually cook and eat your breakfast. It's very important to realize that food is not your enemy; it's your energy source, and you need to feed your muscles and starve your fat.

CALORIES: SHOULD YOU COUNT THEM?

I do not believe in counting every calorie you eat. But I do want you to make sure that you're eating at least 1,000 calories per day. Do not under eat. If your body does not get 1,000 calories per day, then it will conserve fat. When you do this, you will lose scale bodyweight for a while, but then you will start gaining weight at an alarming rate. And all the weight you gain will be fat not muscle.

Remember you want to lose fat—never muscle. Under eating will cause you to cannibalize muscle for energy before you tap into fat. That's true no matter your goal, gender or current bodyweight. Remember the more muscle you have, the more calories you burn.

What follows is a list of breakfast ideas, but do not limit yourself to these. Food choices are completely up to you so long as you stay within the parameters of my portion-size recommendations while adhering to the GL principles.

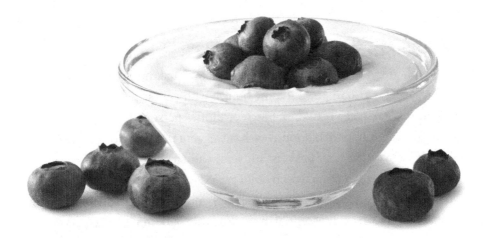

BREAKFAST RECIPES

YOGURT

Plain Greek yogurt 6 oz add 2 oz of any fresh berries you like:
Do not eat the yogurt with the fruit already added. Fresh fruit is better than fruit that has been sitting in yogurt for a few weeks, and fruit versions often contain added sugar.

	Calories:		
6 oz	**0% fat**	**1% fat**	**2% fat**
Chobani	100	n/a	130
Okios	120	n/a	n/a
Stonyfield	80	n/a	140
Wallaby	100	130	170
Fage	100	130	190

Any of these types of yogurt are fine for my program. Again, you don't need to count calories. I'm just showing you how they vary when you include differing levels of dietary fats. Choose the type you like best.

	Calories:
2 oz	
Blueberries	33
Strawberries	19
Raspberries	30
Blackberries	24
Pomegranate seeds	47
Grapes	38
Banana	50
Pineapple	28

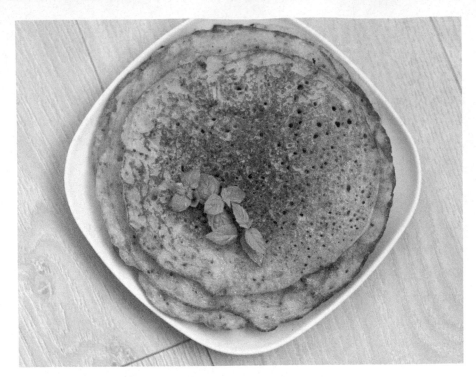

Protein Pancakes

Ingredients:

1 scoop of protein powder (unflavored, 0 sugar)
1 egg
1 spoonful of ground flaxseed
1 teaspoon of vanilla extract
Pinch of cinnamon
Pinch of stevia
Almond milk (optional)
Greek yogurt (optional)

Instructions:

1. Add all the ingredients together.
2. Mix the batter until it reaches desired consistency. If needed, add almond milk (1 spoonful at a time to thin out the mix).
3. Then cook on griddle over low heat, flipping when the top begins to bubble.
4. Top with Greek yogurt or eat plain.

Yogurt Parfait

Ingredients:

1 can of unsweetened pumpkin puree
2 small pears (super ripe)
1 tablespoon of maple syrup
¼ tablespoon of nutmeg
1 cup of 0 fat Greek yogurt
1 cup of rolled oats

Instructions:

1. Blend everything except the yogurt and rolled oats in a food processor.
2. Then place the mixture in the fridge for 30 minutes.
3. Then layer the puree with the yogurt and add the rolled oats on top. *Serves 3*

EGGS

Each large egg contains about 7 g of protein and 13 essential vitamins and minerals. A large egg contains a little more than 200 mg of cholesterol, mostly from the egg yolk, and just over 70 calories. I'm not telling you to eat only one egg; I'm just showing the amount of calories so you know. I want you to eat enough food so you are satisfied and not hungry.

Keep in mind that the calorie count does not include how the eggs and vegetables are prepared. Some options are to use an old skillet so the eggs don't stick, or add canola spray to the skillet.

You can also add olive oil or butter to the skillet, but realize that these add calories and fat, but that may not be negative, depending on how much you're eating for the day. Some people like to cook eggs in their microwave.

To do this:

- coat a microwavable cup with cooking spay;
- pour in your eggs and whatever else you want to add (onions, chopped vegetables, etc.);
- microwave on high for 45 seconds then stir it around and put it back in for another 35 seconds, adjusting the time based on your microwave.

Make sure to watch your eggs the first time you cook them in your microwave! You don't want them to boil over or blow up.

	Calories:
1 Large egg	78
1 Large egg white	17
1 Large hard-boiled egg	78
1 Large hard-boiled egg white	17
1 Egg whites with ½ cup spinach	20
1 Egg with ½ cup spinach	81
1 Egg whites with 2 oz salmon	121
1 Egg with 2 oz salmon	196
1 Egg white with 2 oz mushrooms	30
1 Egg with 2 oz mushrooms	91
1 Egg whites with 2 oz tomatoes	27
1 Egg with 2 oz tomatoes	88
1 Egg white with cheese	178
1 Egg with cheese	236
1 Egg white with broccoli	97
1 Egg with broccoli	36
1 Egg white with eggplant	31
1 Egg with eggplant	123

Healthy Pancakes

Ingredients:

2 eggs
1 medium ripe banana (230 calories)

Instructions:
1. Peel and mash up the banana until its consistency is like thick cream.
2. Then whisk in 2 whole eggs. The mix should look like liquidy eggs, not pancake batter.
3. Take 2 tablespoon of your mix and put it on a hot skillet or non-stick pan.
4. Brown the bottom of the pancake and then flip it over. This should take about 1 minute or so. If it takes longer, then turn up the heat on the stove.
5. Once both sides are golden you are done. You can also add topping like 90% or higher chocolate bits, natural peanut butter or nuts. Some people like to add in ⅛ teaspoon of baking soda to the original mix to make the pancakes fluffier.

Spinach and Cheddar Quiche

Ingredients:

½ cup chopped spinach frozen or fresh
1 egg
½ cup of low-fat milk
⅓ cup of shredded cheddar cheese
A pinch of salt

Instructions:
1. If the spinach is fresh, put in 3 tablespoons of water, cook for 1 min on high then drain. If the spinach is frozen, defrost it and drain out excess water.
2. Then add in the egg, milk, cheese, and salt. Mix it together for 15 seconds.
3. Microwave on high for 3 minutes. Make sure you put a paper towel over the top of the microwavable cup you are using. *Serves 1*

COTTAGE CHEESE

Cottage cheese is packed with protein and essential amino acids. I recommend it after morning workouts because it's naturally high in leucine, which is one of the amino acids that helps build muscle. Vitamin B-12 and calcium are also found in cottage cheese.

	Calories:		
6 oz	**0% fat**	**1% fat**	**2% fat**
Cottage Cheese	123	123	147

2 oz	
Blueberries	33
Strawberries	19
Raspberries	30
Blackberries	24
Pomegranate Seeds	47
Grapes	38
Banana	50
Pineapple	28

Ideas of what to do with cottage cheese:
- Cottage cheese on Ezekiel bread, add slices of avocado or guacamole.
- Cottage cheese on Ezekiel bread, add slices of avocado or guacamole and tomato slices
- Cut 1 banana, put it over 6 oz (0% fat) cottage cheese, and sprinkle ground cinnamon over it.
- 6 oz cottage cheese (0% fat), 10 almonds, 2 oz raspberries

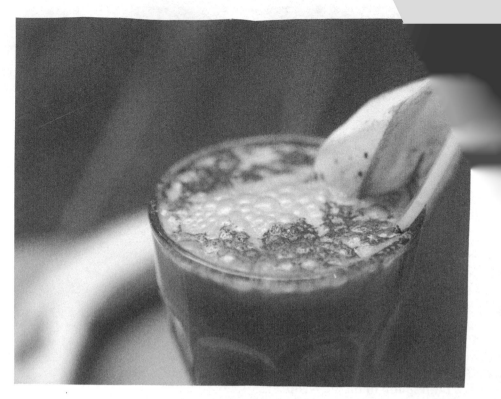

VEGAN BREAKFAST OPTIONS THAT NON-VEGANS WILL LOVE

Chocolate Shake

Ingredients:

1 frozen banana (peel before freezing)
1 tablespoon of peanut butter
2 dates
½ cup of almond milk
1 tablespoon of cocoa
½ teaspoon of Konjac glucomannan powder (optional to thicken your shake)

Instructions:

1. Put the frozen banana, the peanut butter, the dates, almond milk, cocoa and Konjac glucomannan powder in a blender.
2. Blend for 20 seconds and you have your chocolate shake.

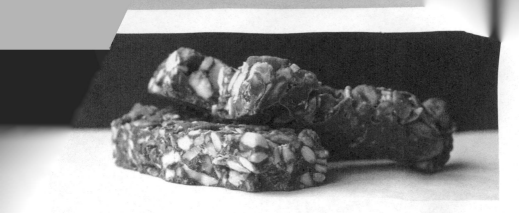

Chocolate Vegan Granola Bar

Ingredients:

1¾ cups of rolled oats

½ cup of chocolate protein powder

1 tablespoon of chia seeds

1 tablespoon of cocoa powder

¼ teaspoon of salt

½ cup of peanut butter

2 tablespoon of maple syrup

½ cup of unsweetened almond milk

2 tablespoons of chopped almonds

2 tablespoons of cacao nibs

Instructions:

1. Preheat oven to 350 degrees.
2. In a medium bowl, combine the oats, protein powder, chia seeds, cocoa powder and salt.
3. In another microwavable bowl, add the peanut butter and maple syrup. Microwave on high for 30 seconds.
4. Stir them together.
5. Then add the milk and stir it all together.
6. Spread the mix into a 9x9 greased pan.
7. Place the almonds and chocolate nibs on the top and press them in.
8. Bake for 15-18 minutes.

This will yield 8 servings that are about 250 calories a serving.

Banana Beet Bowl

Ingredients:
¾ cup of chopped roasted beets
¾ cup of frozen raspberries
½ cup of unsweetened almond milk
1 tablespoon of lime juice
1 scoop of vanilla vegan protein powder
1 tablespoon of flax meal
1 ripe banana
2 tablespoons of sliced almonds (optional for toppings)
¼ cup of any berry (optional for toppings)

Instructions:
1. Place all the ingredients in the blender and blend for 15-20 seconds.
2. Top off the bowl with sliced almonds and ¼ cup of any berry you like and eat it right away.

Quinoa Nut Bowl

Ingredients:
1 cup of unsweetened almond milk
1 cup of water
1 cup of quinoa
2 cups of blackberries or blueberries
⅓ cup of chopped almonds
2 teaspoons of agave

Instructions:
1. Combine almond milk, water and quinoa in a saucepan.
2. Bring to a boil then reduce heat and simmer for 15 minutes.
3. Stir occasionally until most of the liquid is absorbed.
4. Turn off heat and let it stand for 5-10 minutes.
5. Then add in blackberries or blueberries and mix them in. *Serves 4*

Banana Pancakes

Ingredients:
1½ cups oat flour
1 cup almond milk unsweetened
1 very ripe banana

Instructions:
Mix all 3 ingredients in a high-speed blender. Then place the mix on a hot griddle or non-stick pan. Pour in ⅓ of a cup of the batter per pancakes, cook each side till golden brown. You can add in whatever you like, but when these are done the calorie count will be 730 for all the pancakes you made.

Superhero Quick Starts

- Vegan protein shake: Mix the suggested amount of protein powder in with a cup of unsweetened almond milk and 1 banana and your choice of 1 cup of berries (300 calories)

- Apple with 1-2 tablespoons organic peanut butter/almond butter

- Banana with 1-2 tablespoons organic peanut butter/almond butter

- Low-carb cereal (cereals with less than 15 carbohydrates per serving); serve with almond milk or eat dry

- Fruit salad

- Salad for breakfast; use kale and fruit salsa or regular salsa as dressing

- 1 tablespoon of almond butter 95 calories (eat this like a spoon of ice cream)

- 1 slice Ezekiel bread with guacamole (option: squeeze a little lemon on it with chili powder)

- 1 slice of Ezekiel bread with nut butter and ½ sliced banana on top

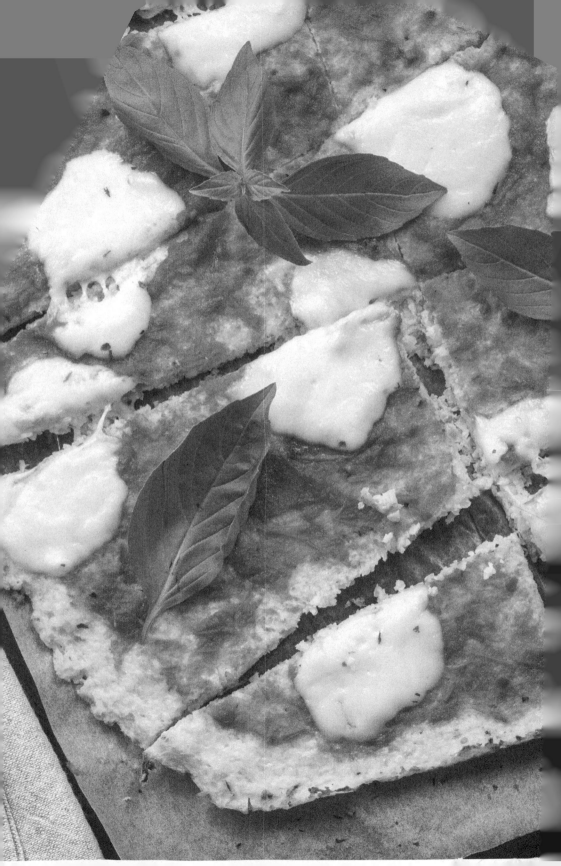

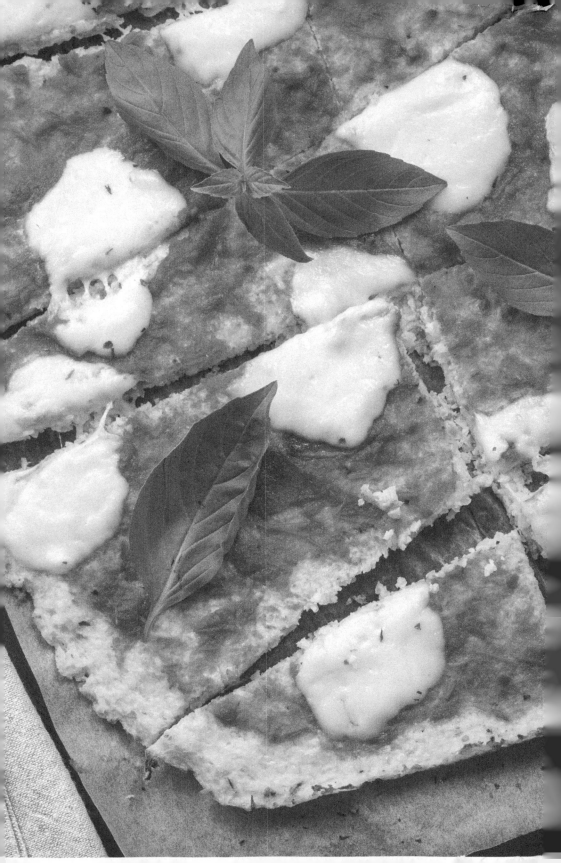

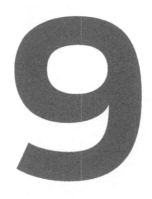

LUNCH & DINNER RECIPES

Healthy, Satisfying Meals

consider lunch and dinner to be interchangeable meals. Some people prefer a large lunch and a small dinner. Other people like a small lunch and a large dinner. That is completely up to you. I also know people who skip breakfast and eat a large lunch and a large dinner. While I don't recommend this, you can still make it work. Everybody's lifestyle is different, so choose the strategy that will help you stay committed to the program.

What follows is a list of recipes and meal options that can be utilized in hundreds of different dishes by mixing and matching proteins with different vegetables. Here's how it works:

- Protein. Start with about 6 oz. of skinless chicken, any kind of fish, turkey, white meat pork, or lean steak.

- Salad. Add a salad with as many greens as you want. They are a "free" food, meaning you can eat as much as you want during your meal. Be aware of the dressing you're adding to your salad. Many salad dressings are surprisingly high in sugar and calories. To avoid heavy dressings, follow my instructions on page 168 to make "Superhero Salad Dressings."

- Veggies. Next add 1-2 cups of any of the vegetables in the nearby chart. To prepare the vegetables, steam, grill or sauté in less than 1 tablespoon of oil or a low-calorie pan spray.

- Dessert. You can eat a piece of fruit or Greek yogurt for dessert if you like, and then you're all set. I personally do this a lot for lunch.

VEGETABLES

Broccoli, cooked
Cabbage, cooked
Spinach
Mushrooms
Cauliflower
Celery, raw
Carrot, raw
Tomato

Green peas
Pumpkin
Peas, frozen
Beets, canned
Asparagus
Zucchini
Bell Pepper
Kale

Brussels sprouts
Green bean
Eggplant
Artichoke
Chard
Cucumbers

A WORD ON FOOD PREP

When cooking chicken always take the skin off first or the fat seeps into the chicken. Many people think they can cook it with the skin on and then take it off, so they are eating skinless chicken. It is skinless but much of the damage is already done during the cooking process.

A lot of my clients tell me they do not have time to really cook anything. To make it easy to have a lunch or dinner on my program you can buy or go out to get lunch or dinner so long as you keep the foods you buy simple, and you talk to your waiter or waitress about how the foods are prepared.

Superhero Salad Dressings

⭐ I prefer using these items for salad dressing: squeezed lemon, salsa, soy sauce, vinaigrette dressings, turmeric tahini dressing, Asian salad dressing (usually sesame), and Greek salad dressing.

Look at the labels for the sugar- and carbohydrate-content for your dressing. A couple of tablespoons of any other type of dressing is fine, but if your salad is bathed in calorie-laden ingredients, you can miss your goal. Choose dressing with less than 1 g of sugar per serving when you're eating your salad as a "free" food. If you're adding more dressing, then check out it's glycemic load.

If you're getting your food to-go at a grocery store or market, then buy about 6 oz of fish, chicken or protein of your choice from the primary protein source list. Purchase pre-cut lettuce at your local market—whatever type you like. Add your protein to this salad, combining with a dressing that contains less than 1 g of sugar.

Choosing different ways to prepare a food makes that same food more interesting and tasty. Try to change it up because boredom can backfire, and then you go for a pizza out of desperation.

But if you want a pizza, I'll teach you how to make my famous cauliflower-crusted pizza. That's my first recipe in this chapter.

Steve's Famous Cauliflower Pizza

Ingredients:

1 package of cauliflower rice (riced cauliflower takes the work out of processing it and cleaning it up after)
2 whole eggs
⅛ cup of almond flour
¼ cup of shredded mozzarella cheese
2 tablespoons of marinara sauce
¼ cup of your favorite cheese

Instructions:

1. Mix all the ingredients in a bowl.
2. Then put down a large piece of parchment paper (not wax paper) over a pizza stone or cookie sheet.
3. Bake on 500 until golden, not black.
4. Then flip over and continue cooking until golden brown.
5. Add 2 tablespoons marinara sauce or diced tomatoes, ¼ cup of your favorite cheese for a pizza.
6. Put back in the oven for 2 minutes or until cheese is melted. Slice up and enjoy. *Serves 2-3 people unless you're me, then it serves 1. A nice twist is to place your salad on top of the pizza, and cut and eat it with a knife and fork.*

You can use my cauliflower crust to add almost anything on top you can think of that fits your meal plan or just consume it like a piece of bread. My crust is very versatile and if you come up with clever ways of using it, please feel free to email me at: atighteru@aol.com.

CHICKEN CHOICES

Americans eat a lot of chicken every week. We toss chicken into salads, eggs, vegetable sautés, soups and even use it as a finger food. Chicken is used in many different cultures in hundreds of different ways, though we're probably the only ones to make chicken "fingers."

Healthy ways of preparing chicken are baked, grilled or simply roasted. Avoid fried chicken. I strongly suggest that you always prepare your chicken skinless. The fat from the skin increases calories unnecessarily in whatever dish you're preparing.

There's a good reason for chicken's popularity: It's a good source of low-calorie protein. Below are facts from the National Chicken Council. Note that these comparisons are for an equal amount of chicken, not a comparison of piece to piece. For instance, the breast portion is about half of a breast, while the meat from the wing is closer to two full wings. In other words, one wing does not have more calories than a chicken breast.

My thought is that the best way to deal with this is to worry less about how many ounces you're eating and focus more on the hand measurements, realizing that chicken breasts provide less fat and calories for that measurement than do drumsticks, thighs and wings.

TYPE OF CHICKEN	CALORIES (per 3 ½ oz)
Skinless boneless breast	165
Skin-on, bone-in breast	197
Skinless drumstick	175
Skin-on drumstick	216
Skinless thigh	209
Skin-on thigh	229
Skinless wing	203
Skin-on wing	290
Whole chicken—meat only	167
Whole chicken—meat and skin	239

Chicken/Quinoa Bowl

Ingredients:
½ cup cooked quinoa
¾ cup shredded chicken (boil chicken then shred)
1 cup steamed vegetables (root preferred)
1-2 tablespoons vinaigrette

Instructions:
1. In a large pot, boil the chicken and then shred it with a fork.
2. (Extra step if quinoa is uncooked. If cooked skip this step.) In a medium-size pot, add 1 cup of water to the ½ cup of uncooked quinoa and cook for 20 minutes.
3. In another medium pot, cook the vegetables in water for about 5-8 minutes.
4. Plate your food and add the vinaigrette on top.

Grilled Chicken Breast Plate

Ingredients:
1 or 2 chicken breasts grilled, depending on their size (remember the palm and first-row-of-knuckles rule)
1 cup steamed broccoli
1 cup grilled eggplant
2-3 cups green salad with dressing (dressing can be salsa, vinaigrette, squeezed lemon, just no more than 1 g of sugar in the dressing)

Instructions:
1. Grill the chicken breast for 5 to 6 minutes per side or until the chicken is fully cooked.
2. Cut up the eggplant and grill it for 3 to 4 minutes on each side.
3. In a medium pot, boil water and add the broccoli. Steam the broccoli for 5 to 7 minutes.
4. In a medium-size bowl, add your greens and the dressing of your choice and toss the salad.
5. Plate your food.

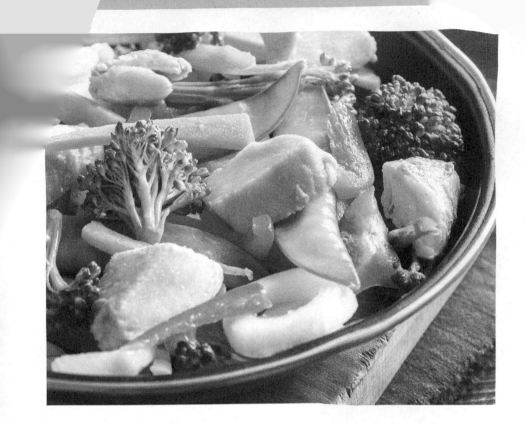

Chicken Stir-fry

Ingredients:
1 chicken breast
2 tablespoons of canola oil
2 cups of mixed vegetables (carrots, broccoli, onion, bell pepper, cauliflower, etc. The amount of each type is based on your preference.)
1 cup of cauliflower rice
2 tablespoons of low-sodium soy sauce

Instructions:
1. Add the canola oil to a nonstick pan or skillet.
2. Stir-fry 1 chicken breast until it is cooked through.
3. Add in 2 cups mixed vegetables and stir the mix until fully cooked.
4. Add the soy sauce to the pan and continue to stir.
5. Cook the cauliflower rice as previously instructed in my cauliflower rice recipe.

Chicken and Cauliflower Casserole

Ingredients:

1 pound of boneless chicken breast

1 package cauliflower rice (you can get a whole cauliflower but you will need to grate it)

1 teaspoon of salt and a pinch of pepper

1 ½ teaspoon of dried parsley

3 tablespoons of heavy cream

1 cup of shredded cheddar cheese

Cooking spray to taste

Instructions:

1. Cut your chicken into cubes.
2. Take a large skillet, add the chicken and cream. Keep heat on medium. Cook chicken until it is lightly browned (could take around 10 minutes).
3. Spray an 8x11 Pyrex dish with your non-stick spray and spread the cauliflower in it, sprinkle the dried parsley, add salt and dash of pepper.
4. Place the chicken on top of the cauliflower then pour the cream over it.
5. Spread the cheddar cheese on top. Bake for 15-20 minutes. *Serves five people.*

Chinese Chicken Salad

Ingredients:

1 chicken breast

1 head of iceberg lettuce or other forms of lettuce

⅛ cup of sliced raw almonds

1 tablespoon of sesame seeds

2 tablespoons of Chinese chicken salad dressing

Instructions:

1. Boil 1-2 chicken breasts till cooked through.
2. Cut up the head of lettuce as thin as you like and put it in bowl.
3. Shred the chicken into strips and spread the chicken over the lettuce.
4. Do the same with the almonds, sesame seeds, and dressing, and mix.

Lettuce-wrapped Chicken

Ingredients:
6 oz chicken breast
3 tablespoons guacamole
3 tablespoons salsa (mild, medium or hot, depending on your taste)
2 lettuce cups
1 tablespoon minced onions

Instructions:
1. Cut the chicken breast into whatever size you prefer.
2. Grill, sauté, etc. once again up to you.
3. Place the chicken evenly in both lettuce wraps, then evenly place the other items on top starting with the guacamole.
4. Wrap it up and enjoy. *Serves two lettuce cups.*

Broccoli Chicken

Ingredients:
½ cup chicken broth
1 tablespoon of low-sodium soy sauce
4 cups broccoli florets
1 clove minced garlic
1 tablespoon of olive oil
1 pound of chicken breast

Instructions:
1. Mix the chicken broth and soy sauce in a bowl.
2. Cook the broccoli in a skillet with the oil until its crispy, then remove from skillet and add it to the bowl of soy sauce.
3. Add chicken to skillet and cook until tender.
4. Then add everything in the bowl to the skillet with the chicken.
5. Bring the whole thing to a boil. Then you are done and ready to eat. *Serves four.*

Non-fried Non-rice Chicken Bowl

Ingredients
1 chicken breast
1 package of cauliflower rice
2 tablespoons low-sodium soy sauce
½ cup of peas
1 tablespoon of lime juice
2 tablespoons of chopped cilantro
1 tablespoon of chopped onions
1 egg

Instructions:
1. Grill 1 chicken breast and cut it into cubes.
2. Microwave the cauliflower rice according to the instructions on the bag.
3. Place the cauliflower in a skillet.
4. Cook on low heat for 2-5 minutes, stirring it frequently to brown a bit, but not burn.
5. Add in the ½ cup of peas.
6. Stir in the low-sodium soy sauce, lime juice, cilantro, and onion.
7. Fry 1 whole egg in pan using cooking spray to line the non-stick pan.
8. Plate your dish by putting the cauliflower in a bowl, adding the chicken, and topping off the dish with the egg.

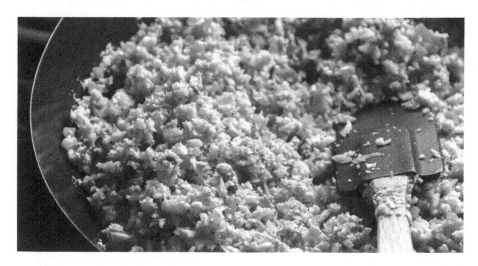

FISH RECIPES

There are many simple ways to prepare fish, including grilling, baking and broiling. Here are several types of fish that you should consider. They're all included in my program, and most of these are primary proteins.

Bass
Striped bass
Black cod/sable
Blue fish
Butter fish
Catfish
Chilean sea bass/Patagonian toothfish
Cod
Flounder
Grouper
Haddock
Halibut
John dory
Mackerel
Mahi mahi
Mullet
Orange roughy
Sablefish
Salmon
Sand dab
Sea bass
Shark
Sole
Sturgeon
Swordfish
Tilapia
Trout
Tuna
Wahoo
Whitefish

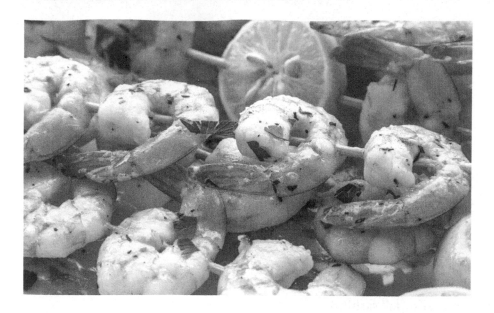

CRUSTACEANS
Crab
Crayfish
Prawn
Lobster
Shrimp

Add two servings of a low-carb vegetable and add a salad and off you go.

On the run? Simply add a 6-oz piece of any fish over a green salad and choose your dressing. I like salsa or a lemon, but any non-sugar added dressing will work. A little hint: if the dressing is creamy, it's probably not your best choice.

More Interesting Fish Dishes

Who likes sushi? I love sashimi, and more and more people around the world are becoming aware of sushi and sashimi. Sashimi is just sushi fish without the rice. Eliminating the rice is a great way to stay on my nutrition program.

I eat lots of fish and vegetables at lunch and dinner. I have sashimi all the time for lunch and dinner, and I don't eat any bread or pasta, which helps keep me from adding bodyfat.

Keep in mind that a single sushi roll has about 1 bowl of rice in it. A bowl of rice has more useless carbs than does a few pieces of white bread. That's not where the problem ends. How is it that the rice is sticky and stays together under sushi and on rolls? SUGAR! Sushi chefs add sugar to the rice to make it sticky rice, which now compounds the issue.

The key is to eat sashimi instead of sushi. I have created and been taught many raw-fish dishes that use no rice. So let me describe a few of these. Hopefully this can spark you into coming up with interesting dishes beyond mine.

Grapefruit Sushi

Ingredients:
4 oz salmon sashimi
4 oz yellowtail sashimi
4 oz blue-fin tuna
12 pieces cooked shrimp
4 grapefruit
Low-sodium soy sauce
Ponzu sauce
Rice vinegar

Instructions:
1. Get 2 bowls, 1 for the grapefruit and grapefruit juice; the other for everything else.
2. Cut the grapefruit in half, squeeze half of them into the bowl, peel the other half of the grapefruit and cut it up into pieces you can eat in 1 bite, place them in the grapefruit juice.
3. Add in 4 tablespoons low-sodium soy sauce, 4 tablespoons ponzu sauce, and 1 drip of rice vinegar.
4. Mix that together.
5. Cut the sashimi and shrimp into ¼ inch blocks and put in second bowl.
6. When done cutting put the fish in the other bowl mix it up and serve.
** **IMPORTANT:** Do not mix the two bowls before you want to eat because after a few minutes the grapefruit starts to cook the fish. *Serves three.*

Spicy Tuna Cucumber Roll

(Note: You can substitute yellow tail, salmon, or any other sashimi if you like.)

Ingredients:

6 oz tuna sashimi

1 large cucumber

2 tablespoons of non-fat mayonnaise

1 tablespoon of sesame seeds

1 tablespoon of Sriracha sauce

2 tablespoons of low-sodium soy sauce

Instructions:

1. Peel the cucumbers, then slice in half the long way and scoop out all the seeds.
2. Chop and mince the block of fish and place in a bowl.
3. Mix in the mayonnaise.
4. Add in a few drops to 1 tablespoon of Sriracha sauce depending on how spicy you want your tuna.
5. Once completely mixed in, take a spoon and scoop the tuna out and put it in the cucumber where the seeds used to be. It will look like a tuna boat.
6. Sprinkle the sesame seeds on top.
7. Drip the low-sodium soy sauce over the rolls.
8. Then, cut the short way into ½ inch pieces. It will look like spicy tuna bites.

I introduced this recipe to my local sushi place. Within a month, they were selling over 100 of my rolls a week.

Grill It!

You can grill your favorite fish, too. Make sure you sear it or cook it all the way through. Cut up double the amount of vegetables than your piece of fish and grill them alongside the fish. I like to sprinkle a tiny amount of salt and pepper on the vegetables. Make a green salad and serve. *Serves 1*

BEEF

Beef is a great food on my program, but I personally only eat beef about once every two weeks. I certainly do not have anything against beef. Growing up in an Argentinian family, beef was a staple. Here are 29 lean cuts of beef with info according to the USDA.

Beef Cuts (a 3-oz serving):	Calories:	Saturated Fat (g):	Total Fat (g):
Eye round roast and steak	144	1.4	4
Sirloin tip side steak	143	1.6	4.1
Top round roast and steak	157	1.6	4.6
Bottom round roast and steak	139	1.7	4.9
Top sirloin steak	156	1.9	4.9
Brisket, flat half	167	1.9	5.1
95% lean ground beef	139	2.3	5.1
Round tip roast and steak	148	1.9	5.3
Round steak	154	1.9	5.3
Shank cross cuts	171	1.9	5.4
Chuck shoulder pot roast	147	1.8	5.7
Sirloin tip center roast and steak	150	2.1	5.8
Chuck shoulder steak	161	1.9	6.0
Bottom round (western griller) steak	155	2.2	6.0
Top loin (strip) steak	161	2.3	6.0
Shoulder petite tender	150	2.4	6.1
Flank steak	158	2.6	6.3
Shoulder center (ranch) steak	155	2.4	6.5
Tri-tip roast and steak	158	2.6	7.1
Tenderloin roast and steak	170	2.7	7.1
T-Bone steak	172	3.0	8.2

Keep it Lean

Beef is high in protein, zinc, iron and vitamin B. Do not fear the fat in beef. Fifty percent of the fat is monounsaturated, which is considered heart healthy.

That said, I only eat lean cuts of meat. I usually grill it, but many people like to broil it. When creating dishes with beef I always group it with low glycemic-load carb foods. I feel it digests better when grouped that way. Higher glycemic-load foods when coupled with beef cause your insulin spike to last longer.

Steak Vegetable Salad with Balsamic Vinaigrette

Ingredients:
Your choice of 6 oz of lean beef
Bowl of green salad
Balsamic vinaigrette

Instructions:
1. Place 5 oz of spring mix baby lettuce or whatever lettuce you like best.
2. Grill or broil 6 oz of your favorite beef; place it on top of the lettuce.
3. Drizzle 2 tablespoons of balsamic vinaigrette over the top of the salad.

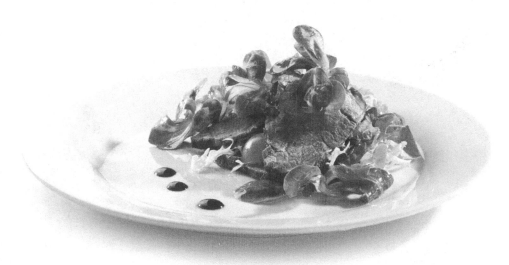

Steak Plate

Ingredients:

6 oz choice of lean beef

Choice of 2 or 3 different side vegetables

Instructions:

1. Grill or broil 6 oz lean cut of beef of your choice.

2. Prepare your choice of vegetables and plate them all together.

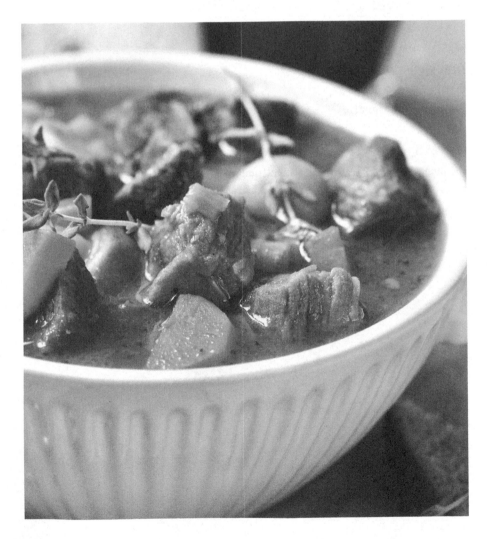

Beef Stew

Ingredients:

2 tablespoons of olive oil
2 pounds of stew meet cut into 1-inch cubes
½ tablespoon of salt
½ tablespoon of ground pepper
4 large carrots cut into ½ inch pieces
4 celery stacks cut ½ inch pieces
2 tablespoons of tomato paste
1 tablespoon of thyme
1 tablespoon of dried rosemary
2 tablespoons of chopped fresh parsley
1 diced onion
3 cups of beef broth

Instructions:

1. Put the burner on medium heat. Using a large pot, add the olive oil and wait for the olive oil to sizzle, which takes about 1-2 minutes after adding it to the pot.
2. Add the meat and stir until all sides of the diced meat are brown.
3. Take the meat out and place it into a medium-size bowl, but try to keep the liquid from the meat and the olive oil inside the pot.
4. Then add the diced onion to the pot and stir for about 5 minutes until it is cooked.
5. Add the diced carrots and celery to the pot and stir them in with the onions for about 2 minutes.
6. Pour in the beef broth and add the meat back into the pot.
7. Add the salt, ground pepper, tomato paste, thyme, rosemary, and fresh parsley to the pot and stir for about 2 minutes.
8. Cover the pot with a lid and reduce the heat to low/simmer for 2 to 2½ hours.
9. Uncover the pot and stir the stew before serving.

The All-American Turkey Burger

A lot of people that I meet with tell me their biggest weakness is burgers and French fries. I know how tempting they are, but you can easily turn a burger into a healthier option. My wife makes the best turkey burgers that are low in fat and sugar.

Ingredients:
1 pound of ground turkey
1 tablespoon of Wellbee's Honey Ketchup
¼ cup of chopped onion
½ teaspoon of salt
A pinch of pepper

Toppings:
1 slice of tomato (optional)
Lettuce

Instructions:
1. Add all the ingredients together in a bowl and knead the ingredients together.
2. Make your patties about 1/3 of an inch thick.
3. Grill your patties on a medium to high heat on an outdoor grill.
4. Grill your burgers for about 5 minutes on each side or until the burger looks cooked.
5. Add your toppings if you would like and enjoy, but do not add a bun to this. That is way too many carbohydrates and unnecessary. *Serves four*

VEGETARIAN DISHES: MEATLESS MAGIC

Veganism is mainstream, and it is here to stay. Because vegan eating is so widespread now, you can get great ingredients to make vegan meals.

Even though I am not vegan I enjoy a whole host of vegan meals and can go days without eating protein that comes from an animal. Many people believe that if they start eating this way they will either wither away or end up eating all carbs and looking puffy. Both of these can happen if you eat empty carbs such as bread, pasta, white rice and white potatoes as your main dishes. But if you take the time to do your homework you can find meals that will create whole proteins that taste great and won't make you fat. I promise.

The following vegan recipes are meals you'll like even if you're not vegan. And, with a slight tweak here or there, you can make it not vegan but still delicious.

Cauliflower has become my secret weapon when it comes to food. This also fits perfectly well when enjoying vegan dishes. I can make it instead of French fries, mashed potatoes, rice, Buffalo wings and even steak.

Cauliflower French Fries

Ingredients:
1 package of cauliflower florets
3 tablespoons of virgin olive oil
1 teaspoon of salt

Instructions:
1. Take a package of cauliflower florets and place them in a Ziploc bag along with 3 tablespoons of virgin olive oil and a teaspoon of salt.
2. Shake the bag up and make sure all the florets are evenly covered in the oil and salt. Let that package of yum sit in the fridge for at least 5 hours.
3. Take the cookie sheet and evenly spread out the cauliflower and put your oven on 350 and cook for 30 minutes.
4. Then turn the cauliflower over and cook for another 30 minutes. The cauliflower should turn dark brown but not black. It should almost look caramelized, guiltless and better than French fries. *Serves three*

Cauliflower Mashed Potatoes

Ingredients:

2½-3 pounds cauliflower florets
1 clove of garlic
1 tablespoon of unsalted butter or olive oil
½ teaspoon of salt
A pinch of pepper

Instructions:

1. Use a medium pot and put all the cauliflower inside it.
2. Fill the pot with water till it covers all the cauliflower.
3. Cover with a lid and bring to a boil. Once it boils reduce the heat to low and cook for around 10 more minutes or until the cauliflower is tender. Then drain.
4. Add the butter or olive oil and spread evenly.
5. Use a high-end blender and pour all the ingredients inside. Put the blender lid on top and blend till smooth.
6. Add salt and pepper and serve like you would mashed potatoes. *Serves four*

Cauliflower Buffalo Wings

Ingredients:

Olive oil spray
¾ cup gluten-free baking flour
1 cup of water
½ teaspoon of garlic powder
A pinch of both salt and ground pepper
2 heads of cauliflower
2 tablespoons of butter
½ cup of hot pepper sauce (optional)
1 teaspoon of honey

Instructions:

1. Mix flour, garlic powder, water, salt and pepper together in bowl. Whisk it all together till the batter is smooth.
2. Now put the cauliflower in the batter until the cauliflower is fully coated. Remove the cauliflower and place on a cookie sheet.
3. Bake in a preheated oven for 20-25 min.
4. In a saucepan, over medium heat melt the butter.
5. Remove from the heat and stir in the honey and optionally the hot pepper sauce until it's smooth.
6. Brush the mix over the cauliflower and bake for another 10 minutes or until browned.
7. Remove the cookie sheet and allow to cool for 10-15 minutes.

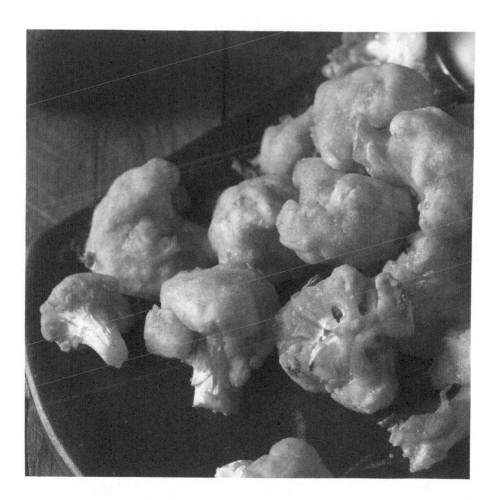

Cauliflower Rice

Ingredients:
1 package of cauliflower rice
1 tablespoon of virgin olive oil

Instructions:
1. Put 1 tablespoon of virgin olive oil in a large skillet on medium heat.
2. Add in the cauliflower rice.
3. Cover with a lid so the cauliflower steams and becomes tender.
4. Cook for 5-8 minutes and now you have guiltless rice.

Jodi's Famous Cauliflower Steak

I kid you not Cauliflower Steak. When I first was introduced to this I was like, "Yeah, right." Now I go crazy for it.

Ingredients:
1 pre-cut cauliflower steak or 1 head of cauliflower, which you will need to cut
½ teaspoon of extra virgin olive oil
Season with salt and pepper

Instructions:
1. Preheat oven to 400 degrees.
2. Place the cauliflower steaks on a baking sheet.
3. Rub in the extra virgin olive oil and season the cauliflower with salt and pepper on both sides of the steak.
4. Cook the cauliflower in the oven for 15 minutes on one side and then turnover the cauliflower to the other side. Let the other side continue to cook for about 15 minutes.

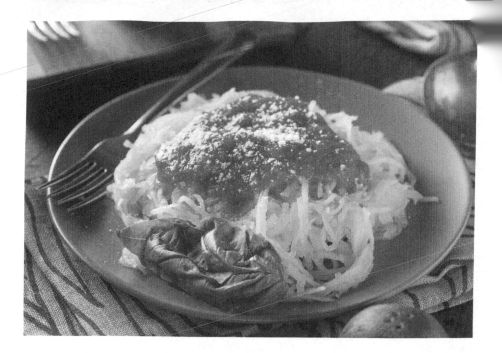

Spaghetti Squash Pasta

Ingredients:

1 spaghetti squash
1 cup of marinara sauce
1 burrata mozzarella ball

Instructions:

1. Preheat the oven to 350 degrees.
2. Cut the squash open lengthwise and scoop out all the seeds.
3. Places the squash cut-side down on a baking sheet and add the tiniest bit of water to the pan to help cook the squash. Let them bake in the oven for about 45 minutes.
4. Take out the squash and use a fork to scrape out the squash spaghetti.
5. Place all the squash that was scraped out into a medium-size bowl.
6. Pour the marinara sauce into the bowl and mix it together with the squash.
7. Plate your spaghetti squash and add your burrata cheese on top (half of the cheese on each plate). *Serves two*

Spaghetti Squash Pasta with Ground Turkey (non-vegetarian version)

Same recipe as above except you add ground turkey to the sauce.

Additional Ingredients:
3 oz. of lean ground turkey

Instructions:
1. Spray canola spray oil in a skillet.
2. Brown the lean ground turkey in it.
3. Drain any liquid that accumulates and add the turkey into the sauce.

Zucchini Spaghetti*

Ingredients:
1 package of zucchini noodles
¼ cup of water
1 tablespoon of olive oil
A pinch of salt
A pinch of pepper
½ cup of fresh chopped tomatoes
2 tablespoons of grated Parmesan

Instructions:
1. Place the olive oil into a skillet on medium heat.
2. Add the zucchini noodles to the oil and stir it for 1 minute.
3. Pour in the water and continue to stir and cook the zucchini for about 6-8 minutes or until the zucchini is softened.
4. Add the salt and pepper to season the zucchini.
5. Place the zucchini into a medium size bowl and mix in the tomatoes and Parmesan.
6. Then plate your dish.

* Make non-vegetarian version by adding ground turkey as prepared above.

Healthy Avocado Toast

Ingredients:
1 slice of Ezekiel bread
½ of a medium-size avocado
½ of a lime
¼ teaspoon of kosher salt

Toppings:
1 sliced tomato (optional)
¼ cup of pomegranate seeds (optional)
1 poached egg (optional)

Instructions:
1. Scoop out the avocado and mush it up in a bowl.
2. Mix the lime juice and salt the avocado.
3. Toast your bread.
4. Spread your avocado on your toast.
5. Optionally, you may add one of the toppings I suggested on top of your avocado spread.

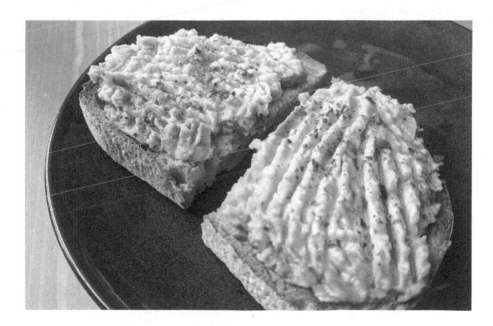

Superhero Soup

⭐ This cabbage soup is another free food that you can add to your other meals, much the same as salads with low- or no-calorie dressings. It's loaded with fiber and very low in calories. You can consume it before, during or after meals so long as you abide by my main rule of not consuming any foods in those five-hour windows between meals.

Keep in mind you can also make up more than one batch of this soup, combining different spices and flavors to provide more variety in your nutrition program.

Ingredients:
1 head cabbage chopped
1 large onions diced
1 can stewed tomatoes (16 oz or so)
½ bunch celery chopped
4-6 large carrots chopped
3 bouillon cubes (beef or chicken, depending on taste)
4-6 gloves garlic (to taste) crushed
1 oz balsamic vinaigrette
1 Tablespoon soy sauce
1 packet onion soup mix
black pepper, basil, chives, cilantro and other spices to taste

Instructions:
1. Chop all vegetables to desired consistency.
2. Cook cabbage and onions adding enough water to cover. If your pot is not large enough to contain all ingredients, add more water as the vegetables cook down.
3. Add bouillon, spices, garlic and other ingredients when you've added the last of the water.
4. Add other vegetables such as carrots, broccoli, green peppers and cauliflower as desired, combining and cooking them to the consistency you desire.

Sweet Potato French Fries

Ingredients:
1 large sweet potato
¼ teaspoon of kosher salt
2 teaspoons of olive oil or canola oil

Dipping Sauce:
1 tablespoon of Wellbee's ketchup (optional)

Instructions:
1. Preheat the oven to 450 degrees.
2. Peel and cut the sweet potato into wedges.
3. In a Ziploc bag, add all the ingredients and shake them together.
4. Spread the wedges out on a baking sheet.
5. Bake the potato for approximately 20 minutes or until the fries look golden brown.

Chinese Food

One of my favorite types of food is Chinese. I know what you might be thinking... Chinese food can be really calorie heavy. However, not all Chinese food is fattening. Just think about a basic Chinese dish. There is always some sort of protein and a vegetable combined in a sauce. Sound familiar?

If you want to make your own Chinese dish, pick one of the following proteins: chicken, beef, pork, or shrimp, and add in a few vegetables of your choice. I often add in some combination of cauliflower, broccoli, string beans, red pepper and mushrooms, but you can add whatever vegetables you like.

Saute the protein and vegetables together in a pan on medium heat with 2 tablespoons of low-sodium soy sauce. To replace the rice, you can either make cauliflower rice or quinoa, both of which I explained how to make earlier in this chapter.

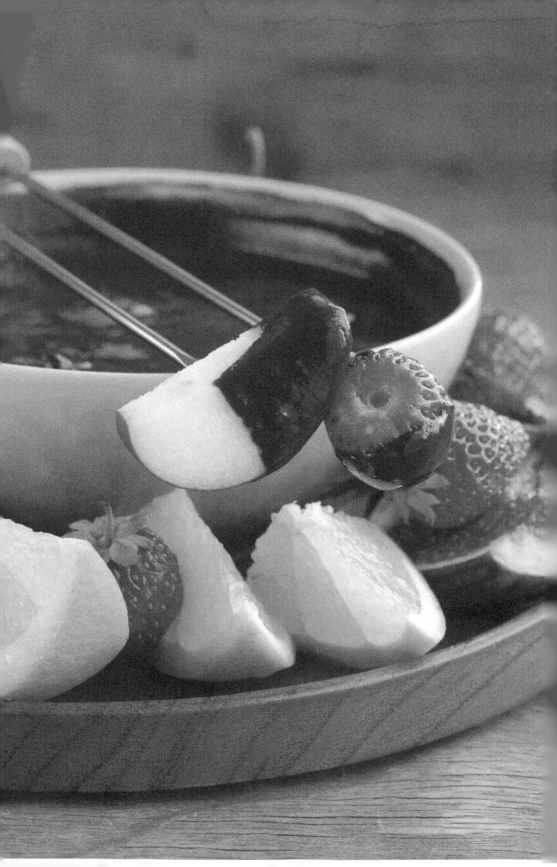

10

GUILTLESS DESSERT RECIPES

Sweet Treats for a Lean Machine

f you have a sweet tooth and that has been your downfall, then this chapter is for you. This is my problem: All day long I do a great job of following my program, but by evening I'm craving something sweet. My two daughters have pointed this out to me several times. They all have the same craving for sweets late in the day, but they also love these healthy dessert options that are on my program. We make them as a family.

Some of these recipes are even my daughters' concoctions. A very simple, yet healthy dessert option is frozen fruit. My favorite fresh fruits to freeze are grapes and blueberries because biting into them tastes like Italian ice. But, you can freeze any fruit you like. This is a great and easy start for eating healthy desserts, but if you want to expand your dessert options, here are a few of my recipes.

Chocolate Fondue

Ingredients:
1 oz of a 90% or higher dark chocolate bar
1 bowl of fruit (any fruit: strawberries, pineapple, melon, etc.)

Instructions:
1. Melt 1 oz of the chocolate bar in the microwave. Don't melt it all the way because it might burn, melt it ¾ of way, which will probably take about 40 seconds on high.
2. Then dip your fruit in it and enjoy a decadent dessert without any guilt. The chocolate has such high fiber that it offsets the moderate amount of sugar. *Serves 1*

Chocolate Protein Pudding

Ingredients:
1 box of sugar-free instant pudding
1 scoop of your favorite plain protein
½ teaspoon of konjac glucomannan powder (optional)
½ cup of the milk of your choice

Instructions:
1. Take the sugar-free instant pudding and add 1 scoop of your protein.
2. Mix it in dry until the protein absorbs into the pudding mix.
3. Add the konjac glucomannan powder to thicken the pudding and add whatever milk you desire. (if you are using almond or rice milk add ½ cup less, or the pudding will have a hard time thickening) *Serves as many as the pudding mix says.*

Banana Ice Cream

Ingredients:
3 frozen bananas
3 tablespoons of your favorite type of milk
2 tablespoons of cocoa nibs (optional)

Instructions:
1. Place the frozen bananas and the milk into a blender.
2. Blend until the mixture looks creamy, about 30 seconds.
3. Fold in the cocoa nibs if you chose to do so, but do not blend them.
4. Empty the mixture into a bread or brownie pan and make sure the mixture is evenly spread across the pan.
5. Freeze for 2 hours. *Serves 3*

Peanut Butter Banana Ice Cream

Ingredients:

3 frozen bananas

3 tablespoons of your favorite type of milk

2 tablespoons of peanut butter

1 tablespoon of cocoa nibs (optional)

Instructions:

1. Place the frozen bananas, milk and peanut butter into a blender.
2. Blend until the mixture looks creamy, about 30 seconds.
3. Empty the mixture into a bread or brownie pan and make sure the mixture is evenly spread across the pan.
3. Freeze for 2 hours.
4. You can additionally add 1 tablespoon of cocoa nibs on top if desired.
   Serves 3

Strawberry Ice Cream

Ingredients:

1 cup of frozen strawberries

3 tablespoons of your favorite type of milk

Instructions:

1. Place the frozen strawberries and the milk into a blender.
2. Blend until the mixture looks creamy, about 30 seconds.
3. Empty the mixture into a bread or brownie pan and make sure the mixture is evenly spread across the pan.
3. Freeze for 2 hours. *Serves 1*

Greek Yogurt Smoothie

Ingredients:
1 cup of Greek yogurt
½ cup of ice cubes
½ of a frozen banana
1 cup of any type of fruit you like in your smoothie (I generally add berries such as raspberries, blueberries, strawberries and blackberries, but you can add anything you would like.)
¼ teaspoon of konjac glucomannan powder (optional)

Instructions:
1. Place all the ingredients into a blender.
2. Blend the ingredients for about 30 seconds or until the fruit is completely blended in and there you have a healthy dessert.

Green Smoothie

Ingredients:
1 cup of fresh spinach
¾ cup of water, coconut water or almond milk (It's up to you!)
1 frozen banana
½ cup of pineapple
½ cup of mango, oranges or apples (Again it is up to you!) This smoothie is great because you can mix different ingredients and see what you like best!

Instructions:
1. Put the spinach and the liquid base you chose into a blender and blend the mixture until it turns into a puree.
2. Then, place the rest of the ingredients into the blender and blend for about 30 seconds or until all the fruit is completely blended.

Final Thoughts:
More Helpful Tips for Better Results

⭐ Here are some of my favorite tips for helping you derive even more success from my nutrition program.

1. Brush your teeth after eating. It's hard to have a sweet tooth with a minty taste in your mouth.

2. Chew sugar free gum if it's not your time to eat but you want something in your mouth.

3. Eat slowly. Let your brain realize its full.

4. Keep food away from where you watch TV, studying, working, etc. If you have to go and get food you are much more likely to skip it than if it's right next to you.

5. If you feel hungry, try drinking a glass of water first (I keep banging this water thing home, because it is crucial to attaining your goal).

6. Don't bring junk food home. Do not have food you should not eat in your house.

7. Out of sight, out of mouth. If you must have junk food in your house, then do not have it laying out in a clear container. Keep it out of sight and out of mind.

8. Don't serve food family style. Plate it. Eat it. No seconds.

9. Drink 12 oz of water first thing when you wake up.

10. Never eat at least 2 hours prior to any workout if you plan on burning fat for energy. (Your body might take up to 2 weeks to get used to converting fat quickly for energy, but keep working at it. Most people get used to this in less than a week).

The Ultimate Banana Smoothie

Ingredients:
1 frozen banana
1 ½ cup of ice
½ cup of vanilla almond milk, unsweetened
¼ teaspoon of konjac glucomannan powder

Instructions:
1. Place all the ingredients into a blender.
2. Mix in a high power blender for approximately 45 seconds, or until the smoothie is thick, but still smooth.

Acai Bowl

Ingredients:
1 frozen banana
1 package of unsweetened acai puree packets (You can buy acai berries at Trader Joe's or other specialty grocery stores)
¼ cup of frozen blueberries
¼ cup of frozen blackberries
¼ cup of frozen raspberries
¼ cup of frozen strawberries
½ cup of non-fat milk or unsweetened almond milk
3 tablespoons of granola
1 tablespoon of honey or agave

Instructions:
1. Put the banana, acai berries, blueberries, blackberries, raspberries, strawberries and milk into a blender.
2. Mix the ingredients on high for about 30 seconds or until the fruit is completely blended.
3. Place your mixture into a bowl and add the granola and honey/agave on top.
4. You can add a few berries on top if you would like as well.

Chocolate Covered Fruit

Ingredients:

3 oz of a 90% or higher dark chocolate bar
Any type of fruit. Some of my favorites for this are: strawberries, melon,
pineapple and apples, but you could use any type of fruit.

Instructions:

1. Melt the chocolate bar in the microwave for 40 seconds on high. Don't melt it all the way because it might burn; melt it ¾ of the way.
2. Then dip your favorite fruit into the chocolate and place it on a plate.
3. Place your chocolate covered fruit into the fridge for about an hour or until the chocolate has fully hardened.

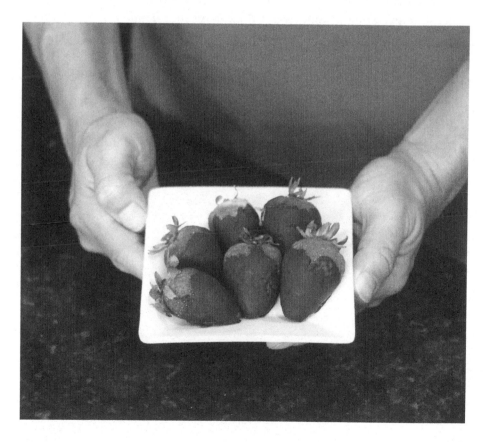

SUPERHERO STORY: THE LAST WORD

You've probably been trying to figure out this whole nutrition Rubik's Cube your entire life. Many of you have gone through several different eating plans and were excited about finally realizing your goal, only to end up disappointed and frustrated when you returned to regular eating patterns. Then you regained the weight you lost and felt even worse than when you started.

To all of you out there with this experience, I share your anguish. I have spent my personal and professional life trying to find the perfect nutrition plan to get your body toned with maximum definition. Once I achieved this program for myself, I perfected it with my clients. Now I am sharing it with you.

As I mentioned earlier, I could make you count calories, but very few people end up doing this successfully for longer than a few days. But when you eat three times a day and leave at least five hours between meals, the human body becomes a fat-burning machine during most of its waking day. Just remember that when it comes to portions, *trust your hand.*

This strategy gives you the leeway to eat a little more if you are still hungry, preventing you from coming to resent your nutrition program after you've hit some "magic" number of calories. Make this program yours by adding innovative choices within your parameters I've explained, enjoy what you are eating, and never allow yourself to feel hungry or deprived. You'll still be able to burn all your excess bodyfat. And, finally, you'll feel comfortable in your own skin and let your true self shine without being self-conscious ever again.

Love your body—you own it!

ACKNOWLEDGMENTS

First and foremost, I'd like to thank all of my clients for their dedication and hard work. Many of my clients have been with me since the beginning and have supported—and continue to support—my vision of health and fitness. This includes Donald and Mickey Mann, Dennis Weiss, David and Sandy Brokaw, the Dugan Family, the Hughes Family, Elizabeth Spellman, Sandra Stern, Carl Beverly, Sandie Wiesenthal, Evelyn Desser, Deborah Goldfarb, Deborah Koniak-Griffen and many others.

I'd like to give a special "thank you" to Rachel Katz, Bryan Arceo, Kennedy Meek, Teresa Conrad, Nick Schaeffer, Willy Rosenfeld, Ben Villers, Auston Ashworth, and Stevi Perry for being the best trainers I know.

Many professional and Olympic athletes have trusted me with their workout regimes, and I have always taken great pride in that. Actors, actresses, directors, and producers have hired me to give the characters they want portrayed a certain look that is vital to the success of their projects. Nobody wants to see a superhero that does not look perfect.

Next, I'd like to thank my family: My wife Jodi and two daughters Carli and Taylor for always encouraging and supporting me no matter how much time it takes to get my projects completed. Jodi once said to me, "Start one project and complete it; don't start several and get nothing done." That one sentence has been the main mantra of my professional life.

I'd also like to thank BuzzFeed and other media entities, including *The Today Show*, *Extra*, and *Entertainment Tonight*. They've helped me get my message out to the world, and one them may be the reason you're holding this book in whatever form—print or digital—right now.

Finally, I'd like to thank the team who put this book together from conception, drafting, layout to publication. These include: Kimberly Richey (designer and photographer), Jim Schmaltz (editor), Steven Stiefel (co-writer and publishing coordinator), Michael Duran (front cover graphics), Carli Zimelman (recipe contributor), Syd Scrivano (cataloger & illustrator), Clint Gage (first-draft editor), Josh Dassa (first-draft reader), Kennedy Meek (photographer), Nick Sage (photographer), Taylor Zimelman (social media director), Ted Bear, for being my best running partner.

This book could not have been possible without the contribution of all these people.

- Steve Zim

97293029R00116

Made in the USA
Middletown, DE
04 November 2018